Planning a For

GW00371976

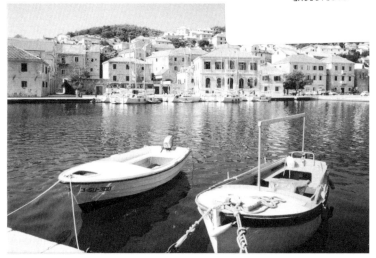

Information for yachts visiting
the Mediterranean and the Black Sea

**A companion volume, Planning a Foreign Cruise C1,
contains information regarding countries in Northern Europe**

Compiled from various sources
Revised by Jeffery Kempton and Robin Sjöberg

Published jointly by:

Cruising Association
CA House
1 Northey Street
Limehouse Basin
London E14 8BT
Tel: 0171 537 2828
Fax: 0171 537 2266
Email: www.cruising.org.uk

Royal Yachting Association
RYA House
Romsey Road
Eastleigh, Southampton
Hampshire SO50 9YA
Tel: 01703 627400
Fax: 01703 629924
Email: admin@rya.org.uk

CONTENTS

			Page
Chapter	1	General Information	3
Chapter	2	Gibraltar	9
Chapter	3	Spain	11
Chapter	4	France and Corsica	14
Chapter	5	Italy	18
Chapter	6	Slovenia/Croatia/Montenegro	21
Chapter	7	Albania	24
Chapter	8	Malta	25
Chapter	9	Greece	28
Chapter	10	Cyprus	33
Chapter	11	Turkey	36
Chapter	12	The Black Sea	41
Chapter	13	Syria	43
Chapter	14	Lebanon	44
Chapter	15	Israel	45
Chapter	16	Egypt	47
Chapter	17	Libya	49
Chapter	18	Algeria	49
Chapter	19	Tunisia	50
Chapter	20	Morocco	52
Chapter	21	Rhine-Danube Link	53

Should visitors find that regulations or practices differ from those described in these pages, information would be gratefully received and should be addressed to the Cruising Association or to the Royal Yachting Association.

The publishers wish to record their appreciation of the assistance received in the preparation of this booklet from many people, including embassies and tourist offices of the countries concerned, Cruising Association Honorary Local Representatives and numerous cruising yachtsmen who have written of their experiences.

Some regulations are more strictly applied than others. Where there is a difference of opinion, the official line has always been quoted. Local interpretation may be more or less rigid.

Whilst every effort has been made to ensure the accuracy of this publication, neither the compilers, nor the Cruising Association nor the Royal Yachting Association or any of their officers accept any responsibility for the results of any errors or omissions.

March 1999.

1
GENERAL INFORMATION

PURPOSE

This booklet has been written to help a yachtsman plan a cruise to the most widely visited Mediterranean countries, and to comply with their regulations and requirements. It covers the countries bordering the Mediterranean and the Black Sea.

A companion volume deals with countries bordering the Baltic, North Sea and the Atlantic coasts of Europe.

Most of the information applies to boats owned by private individuals. More detailed advice will be needed by yachtsmen who plan:
– to base their boat outside the EU.
– to import their boat permanently into a country outside the EU.
– to cruise in a company-owned yacht.
– to offer their boat for charter or use it for any other commercial purpose.

This advice should be obtained directly from the country concerned. A list of addresses that can be used as starting points is given at the end of each chapter. Allow plenty of time.

A section has been devoted to non-European Union (EU) residents visiting the EU. It is intended to help in the planning of the visit but it is stressed that different interpretation is placed on EU regulations in different member states and early consultation with individual member states authorities is essential for peace of mind and to avoid misunderstanding.

CUSTOMS

Pleasure craft arriving in and departing from the EU are subject to Customs regulations. These are described below.

A vessel owned by an European Union resident is entitled to free movement throughout the EU, with no time limits, as long as the vessel has VAT paid status within the EU. However, it should be noted that some countries may enforce local regulations once a boat has been there for six months.

Vessels owned by non-EU residents and registered outside the EU are entitled to tax free temporary importation into the EU for six months. Longer periods may be granted for laying up or repair but Customs must be contacted to arrange this concession. See non-EU residents section.

CUSTOMS PROCEDURES

Departure from any EU port direct to any other EU port:
no action required.

Arrival in any EU port direct from any other EU port:
no action required unless there are non-EU residents on board, or anything to declare such as firearms.

Departure from any EU port direct to any non-EU port:
inform Customs – in UK complete Form 1331. This applies to all vessels.

Arrival in any EU port direct from any non-EU port:
fly flag Q at 12 mile limit. Contact Customs – they will tell you what to do. Be prepared to prove VAT status of vessel.

Outside the EU practices vary; they are described in the corresponding chapters. If in doubt, skippers should:
– fly flag Q on first entering territorial waters
– if not boarded by Customs on arrival at their first port, present the ship's papers to the nearest Customs office.

See non-EU residents section for details of countries inside and outside the VAT area of the EU.

IMMIGRATION AND HEALTH

It is the responsibility of the owner or skipper:
– to report any cases of suspected infectious diseases.
– to ensure that any non-EU passport holder obtains permission to land.

Customs officers often act for their country's immigration and health authorities but in other places it may be necessary to visit several offices. The cooperation of every yachtsman is required to keep rabies out of those areas of Europe that remain rabies free. The regulations on importation and quarantine of animals must be respected.

Rules exist for transporting animals from one country to another even within the EU and vessels carrying animals must ensure they familiarise themselves with the individual country's rules.

FLAGS

A yacht abroad should wear the national ensign of her country of registration. (British yachtsmen should be aware that the blue ensign may be misunderstood.)

A courtesy ensign of the country being visited should be flown from the starboard yardarm. This is the maritime flag of the country visited.

WEATHER FORECASTS

NAVTEX operates in most of the area of this booklet producing written forecasts and navigational warnings in English.

Navarea II – East Atlantic (48°27'N-6°00'S) – may be received in the extreme Western Mediterranean.

Navarea III – Mediterranean and Black Sea - may be received in the Eastern Mediterranean and Black Sea. The stations at Toulon, Valencia (Cabo de la Nao) and Tarifa are operational. Rome, Cagliari and Augusta are testing but reported as unreliable. Coverage west of Italy is still unreliable although scheduled as operational.

NAVIGATION – LORAN C AND GPS
LORAN C

There are no Loran C transmissions in the Mediterranean or the Black Sea as at January 1999, but it is hoped that these will be reinstated as host nations take on responsibility for their own transmitters.

GPS

The datum point for GPS is WGS 84. Most charts are based on other datums and therefore there are differences in Lat and Long positions of up to 1.5M. It is essential to program GPS or any other electronic navigator to the datum of the chart in use, or make corrections for datum differences if this is not possible.

SHIP'S PAPERS

These typically comprise:
- a registration document. This must be the original, not a photocopy.
- evidence of marine insurance
- the ship's radio licence

Each of these is considered in more detail below:

There are two methods of registering a British yacht.

Full registration under Part 1 of the Merchant Shipping Act is open to all vessels whose owner is established in Britain. (It is the only registration open to company-owned yachts.) It involves measurement, which can be through the RYA for craft less than 24m long. Application forms can be obtained from the Registrar of British Shipping and Seamen, PO Box 165, Gabalfa, Cardiff CF4 4UX. Telephone: 01222 768226. Vessels registered on the Part 1 Register without specified renewal date, need to renew their registration every five years beginning as follows:

Year of build	Date for renewal
Before 1950	11 Jan - 31 March 1999
1950 - 70	1 Jan - 31 Mar 2000
1971 - 75	1 Jan - 31 Mar 2001
1976 - 89	1 Jan - 31 Mar 2002
1990 - 94	1 Jan - 31 Mar 2003

If year of build is unknown renew as soon as possible.

The Small Ships Register provides a simpler and cheaper form of registration for pleasure craft under 24m long owned by UK or Commonwealth citizens ordinarily resident in the UK. Registration lasts five years or until a change of ownership, if earlier. SSR is obtained from the Registrar of Shipping and Seamen, PO Box 165, Cardiff, CF4 5FU, Tel: 01222 768206.

The SSR does not record a vessel's tonnage and this has caused difficulties where dues are calculated on tonnage. On inland waters of mainland Europe it is necessary to have a boat's registration number visible on both sides in letters and numbers 150mm high.

- Marine insurance is obviously prudent; policy documents are increasingly demanded in European countries. It is essential that territorial cruising limits are extended as necessary before the voyage is undertaken and then rigidly observed.
- A Radio-Telephone Ship Licence is required for every yacht with R/T equipment installed.

For British registered vessels it can be obtained from: Wray Castle, Ship Radio Licencing, PO Box 5, Ambleside, LA22 0BF. Tel. 015394 34662, Fax. 015394 34663. This licence is not transferable between owners, and must be renewed if the vessel is sold.

It is necessary to register with an accounting authority if you wish to make link calls or use other radio services for which a charge is made when outside the UK. Yacht Transfer Debit (YTD) is used for these services within the UK (not in the Channel Islands). BT offer accounting authority services. Details can be obtained from GB14; Air, Nautical & Maritime Billing, PP 03A26, -Delta Point, 35 Wellesley Road, Croydon CR9 27Z To arrange a contract Tel:0181 666 7694.

A VHF transmitter may only be used under the supervision of a person holding a VHF Operators Certificate of Competence.

The River Rhine

Action when on the River Rhine in: THE NETHERLANDS, FRANCE, GERMANY, LUXEMBOURG and SWITZERLAND. These are known as the Rhine Countries where a new radio system known as ATIS is demanded for boats based on the Rhine. Sea going vessels are exempt from fitting the special radio equipment but are required to use 1 watt transmission power on all channels except Ch 16 and to use their ship's name and call sign each time they transmit. In addition VHF Ch 6, 8 and 72 may be used for personal messages. These requirements are in addition to the compulsory listening watch on local operational channels.

When sailing between EU countries it is suggested that evidence of VAT-paid status of the vessel is carried. This appears to be particularly important in Spain and Greece. This evidence could be any of the following options:

a) The original VAT receipt received at the time of purchase.

b) The VAT receipt for subsequent payment on import or at the outset of the Single Market.

c) The Customs acceptance of relief from VAT, i.e. on change of residence from outside the EU. UK Customs Notice 8 has the details.

d) Proof that the vessel was taken into use prior to 1 January 1985 (1987 for Austrian, Finnish and Swedish vessels) and was lying in the EU on 1 January 1993 (January 1995 for Austrian, Finnish and Swedish vessels).

e) Acceptance by your national Customs authority that the vessel is of Tax Paid status. Note, if the vessel was in Temporary Importation on 1 January 1993 the Customs authority of that country must issue the documentation.

If a Verey pistol, Mark I miniflare or Nico signal flare system is carried, the original of the Firearms Certificate must be produced and the equipment declared when any border, including any EU border, is crossed. A strongbox must be provided on board. The certificate is obtained from the Police. Flares, other than those mentioned above, do not need firearms certificates.

RECREATIONAL CRAFT DIRECTIVE (RCD)

This came in to force on 16 June 1998. Any boat taken into use in the European Economic Area (EEA) which comprises EU + Norway and Iceland, must now be compliant with the essential requirements of this directive. Vessels built in the EEA before this date or used in the EEA before this date are exempt. Visiting vessels are also exempt. The RYA can supply an information sheet on how to seek compliance.

PERSONAL PAPERS

These typically comprise:

– Passport (with appropriate visas if required) should be valid for at least 6 months longer than the planned visit.

– International Certificate of Competence (ICC).

– Radio-Telephone Certificate of Competence.

In addition, some form of personal health insurance is prudent.

Each of these is considered in more detail below:

– Every crew member must have a valid passport and any necessary visas. Passports are not required by UK citizens visiting the Republic of Ireland.

– Several European countries now require

yachtsmen to have some evidence of their ability. For residents in the UK an appropriate document is the International Certificate of Competence, obtainable from the RYA on completion of a test or to holders of the following practical qualifications; RYA Day Skipper, Coastal Skipper, Yachtmaster or National Powerboat Certificate Level II. Applicants for ICCs for inland waters are required to pass a test of the CEVNI rules.
– A Radio-Telephone Certificate of Competence must be held by someone on board (not necessarily the skipper) before the equipment can be used. Application for examination may be made to the RYA.
– Health insurance policies should be examined to ensure that water-based activities are not excluded.

In every case the original document, not a photocopy, must be carried.

UK yachtsmen can obtain reciprocal emergency National Health cover in other EEA countries on production of Form E111, obtainable from UK Post Offices. An associated booklet gives details of the cover available in EEA countries.

ROAD VEHICLE PAPERS

The papers required when taking a boat abroad on a trailer typically comprise:
– the vehicle registration document
– International Driving Licence (outside the EU)
– evidence of insurance for boat and trailer
– The Insurance Green Card is required in most countries and should always be carried. Some countries also require separate cover for a trailer. Your insurer can advise.
– Some form of breakdown and recovery insurance, to cover the trailer as well as the car, is prudent.
– In most European countries, the overall length of vehicle and trailer may not exceed 18m, width 2.5m. Exceptions are indicated in the relevant chapters.
– AA and RAC will provide information and documentation for specific countries.

LOCAL LAWS

Laws vary from country to country – as does the treatment of offenders. A hobby like bird-watching can be misunderstood, especially near military installations.

Copies of local regulations must sometimes be carried on board, e.g. on French inland waterways the carriage of the Inland Water Signals and Regulations (CEVNI) is required. It is contained in the RYA Book of EuroRegs, available from the RYA, price £5 plus £1 postage.

Drug offences are now punishable by massive fines, confiscation of the yacht and long imprisonment; do not carry parcels through Customs for anyone.

CONSULAR ASSISTANCE

British Consulates exist to help British citizens abroad to help themselves. On arrival in a foreign country it is sensible to note the address and telephone number of the local British Embassy, High Commission or Consulate (see the local telephone directory or ask at the Tourist Information Office). A Consul's resources and the help he can give are limited.

If necessary he can:
– issue an emergency passport
– advise on how to transfer funds
– advise on procedures in case of death or accident
– contact British Nationals who have been arrested
– tell you about organisations who can trace missing persons
– cash a small sterling cheque supported by a banker's card
– possibly, as a last resort, make a loan towards repatriation to the UK.

He cannot:
– get you out of prison
– give legal advice
– investigate a crime
– get you a work permit
– pay your bills.

It is sensible to ensure that, in case of disaster, every crew member has sufficient money to buy a ticket home from the furthest point likely to be reached on the cruise.

DUTY-FREE STORES

Yachts planning to voyage beyond the Elbe (actually the north bank of the R. Eider) or Brest are permitted to embark stores duty free in the UK. It is necessary to provide a suitable locker into which the stores can be sealed by a Customs officer until the yacht has left UK waters. The value of this concession to a yacht making a coasting voyage is limited because most countries allow only the normal tourist allowance to be withdrawn from the sealed store whilst the yacht is in their territorial waters. It is necessary to make a written application to Customs who may make a charge for their services. Customs point out that this is not a statutory entitlement but rather a concession that they allow.

It is permissible to import unlimited quantities of alcohol, scent and cigarettes bought tax paid in one EU country into another EU country as long as they are for personal use. Keep the receipt to prove tax status.

PUBLICATIONS

In each of the following chapters there is a list of publications likely to be useful to yachtsmen visiting the country concerned. Of general interest are:

Mediterranean Almanac 1999-2001 (Imray)
Marina Guide Mediterranee, Spain, France, Corsica (Vetus)
Mediterranean Cruising Handbook *Heikell* (Imray)

ADDRESSES

Most of the publications referred to are available from the following chandlers or bookshops:

Kelvin Hughes, 142 The Minories, London EC3 1NH (0171 709 9076) Fax: 0170 481 1298.

Capt. O.M. Watts, 7 Dover Street, Piccadilly, London W1X 3PJ (0171 493 4633) Fax: 0171 495 0755.

Stanfords, 12/14 Long Acre, London WC2E 9LP (0171 836 1321) Fax: 0171 836 0189.

London Yacht Centre,13 Artillery Lane, London E17LP (0171 247 2047) Fax: 0171 377 5680

Warsash Nautical Bookshop, 6 Dibles Road, Warsash, Southampton SO31 9HZ (01489 572384) Fax: 01489 885756.

Dubois, Phillips & McCallum Ltd, Mersey Chambers, Covent Garden, Liverpool L2 8UF (0151 236 2776) Fax: 0151 236 4577.

Most of the foreign publications mentioned can also be obtained from these bookshops, but they are usually cheaper in their country of origin.

An up-to-date list of Agents for British Admiralty Charts is given in the small craft edition of Notices to Mariners, obtainable from chandlers or the RYA.

NON-EU RESIDENTS VISITING THE EU

The European Union has the following member states:

Austria	Germany	The Netherlands
Belgium	Greece	Portugal
Denmark	Ireland	Spain
France	Italy	Sweden
Finland	Luxemburg	United Kingdom

Temporary importation (TI) into these countries is only available to vessels
a) registered outside the EU, and
b) owned by non-EU residents.

Once a person is resident for more than six months in any twelve months in the EU he becomes an EU resident and is no longer entitled to TI. In theory therefore a visitor to the EU from the USA or Australia ceases to be entitled to TI six months after entering any part of the EU, travel within the EU counting as though one remains in a single country of residence. The initial period may be extended for bona fide reasons, e.g.
a) if the boat is laid up and unused,
b) if the boat is undergoing refit or repair,
c) if the owner leaves the EU.

In practice the authorities in member states will almost certainly extend TI for bona fide non-EU visitors to a maximum of about three years, but only by relatively short periods each time, typically six months. It is vital therefore for a visitor to make formal contact with Customs authorities as soon as possible, in each country, to ascertain what rules will be applied. As non-EU residents are required to be notified to immigration whenever an EU border is crossed this is the obvious time to make this formal contact. It may be useful to note those countries, or parts of member states, which are outside the EU VAT area, which may be useful if TI is withdrawn and a vessel chooses to leave the EU. A vessel under TI may not be sold, hired or lent to a non-entitled person. The following are close to the EU but not part of it, some have time limits for TI:

Russia	Lithunia
Poland	Slovenia
Norway	Croatia
Malta	The Channel Islands
Turkey	The Azores
Estonia	Gibraltar (EU but outside
Latvia	Customs zone)

In the past, customs officials in France, particularly on the Atlantic coast, have applied the 6 months in 12 rule very harshly. Visiting vessels have been subjected to very high fines and instant expulsion from France. It is now thought that France permits TI for 2 years but no confirmation is available.

Relief from VAT is available in certain cases of change of residence from outside the EU to inside. UK Customs Notice 8 has details.

CERTIFICATES OF COMPETENCE

Compliance with the rules of one's own flag state, i.e. the state of registry of the vessel, is the normal requirement in coastal waters of other countries. In practice some countries are so used to demanding Certificates of Competence that officials believe they are a legal requirement and will delay vessels where the skipper cannot prove competence. On inland waters it is a matter for that country and some countries do demand Certificates of Competence from all or certain vessels on their inland waters. The various chapters give guidance on this matter. It is therefore wise to arm oneself with some form of Certificate of Competence for navigation in the areas covered in this booklet. Ideally the certificate should be issued by the Government of the skipper's state of residence, but almost any proof of competence is usually accepted, particularly if it includes a photograph, is written in the language of the country visited and is stamped by an identifiable authority. Any new issue of ICC or renewal of an old ICC will now require a written test on the CEVNI rules if the inland waters box is to be ticked.

8

2
GIBRALTAR
(Member of European Union but outside VAT area)

GENERAL INFORMATION

The number of yachts calling at Gibraltar grows year by year and the facilities available to yachtsmen are also increasing. The two original marinas, Sheppards and Marina Bay, have both increased the available moorings, and there is a new marina development, Queensway Quay, inside the harbour. It is also possible for vessels to anchor to the north of the airport runway, but this entails a long trip in the dinghy to reach the shops.

Gibraltar has much to offer the visitor in terms of historic interest, and the Government of Gibraltar is trying hard to promote tourism, consequently entry formalities are fairly relaxed.

Although Gibraltar has its own sterling notes, British notes can be obtained from the banks. Both are legal tender.

Gibraltar has its own airport with direct flights on most days to the UK and Tangier.

Tel. code from the UK: 00 350
Tel. code to the UK: 00 44

ENTRY BY SEA

On arrival skippers should report to the Customs reception berth next to the Shell refuelling station on the starboard side of the approach to the two older marinas. Queensway Quay has its own clearance facility.

CUSTOMS

All items to be brought in duty free must be declared.
1. Upon arrival you are required to supply a crew list in triplicate.
2. To obtain clearance to go ashore travel documents, e.g. passports and, if appropriate, visas are required.
3. Any crew member or passenger intending to reside ashore during the time the vessel is in port must report to the Immigration Control Office, Waterport (0930 - 1300 Mon - Thurs. 1530 - 1700 Fri).
4. If any person on board has employment in Gibraltar, it must be reported to the Immigration Control Office.
5. Before leaving, report time and date of departure to the Immigration Control Office.
6. Immigration control must be advised of any guest residing aboard.

DUTIABLE STORES

Duty free liquor and tobacco may be readily obtained from any wine and spirit merchant on leaving Gibraltar.

ENTRY BY ROAD

The frontier with Spain is fully open, although sporadic problems continue. Short stay trailed craft should have no difficulty in entering Gibraltar provided that the regulations for bringing a boat into Spain have been met (see chapter on Spain).

TEMPORARY IMPORTATION

There is no duty payable on the importation of a yacht into Gibraltar if the owner is not classified as a resident. A resident, for these purposes, is defined as a person who has stayed, or will stay, in Gibraltar for an average of six months or more per year over a period of three years previous to, or subsequent to, the date of importation. However, this rule is interpreted by the Customs authorities to mean that after a continuous stay of eighteen months, or aggregated in a period of less than three years, duty becomes payable. This period may be extended at the discretion of the Collector of Customs. The rate of duty is 12% of the yacht's value at the time of importation.

Gibraltar is part of the EU but outside the EU VAT area. Items being sent out of Gibraltar for repair must first be cleared with Customs and upon return be clearly marked -spares in transit.

DOCUMENTATION OF VESSEL

It is not essential for a yacht to be registered in order to visit Gibraltar, but it is a requirement for Gibraltar based yachts visiting local Spanish ports. If the skipper of the yacht is not the owner then he should have a document, in English and Spanish, authorising the use of the vessel.

CHARTERING

Two charter companies operate in Gibraltar, Enterprise Sailing (01491 572497) and International Charter Centre (01703 455069). Both advertise in British yachting magazines.

FUEL, STORES AND REPAIRS

Petrol and diesel can be obtained at reduced duty rates at the Shell refuelling berth which is adjacent to the Customs reception berth.

Queensway Quay will arrange fuel delivery to the marina cheaper than that available from Shell or Esso.

Exchange or refill of gas bottles is difficult unless these are Spanish bottles and fittings. There is a plentiful supply of English goods at Safeway, close to the marinas. Excellent and comprehensive yacht repair services are available.

WEATHER FORECASTS

Available in English on 1458kHz at 0645, 0730, 1230, and 2359 local time.

PUBLICATIONS

Admiralty Mediterranean Sea Pilot Vol 1
North African Pilot (Imray).

USEFUL ADDRESSES

Gibraltar Information Bureau, National Tourist Office, 179 The Strand, London WC2R 3DT. Tel: 0171 836 0777

Royal Gibraltar Yacht Club, Queensway. Tel: 350 78897.

Sheppard's Marina, Waterport. Tel: 350 77183/75148 Fax: 350 42535

Gibraltar Tourist Office, Cathedral Square. Tel: 350 79336.

Principal Immigration Officer, Waterport, Marina Bay Complex Ltd, PO Box 373 Tel: 350 73300 Fax: 350 78373 (1998)

Queensway Quay Marina, PO Box 19, Ragged Staff Wharf. Tel: 350 44700 Fax: 350 44699

Gibraltar Chart Agency,
4 Bayside Road, Gibraltar.
Tel/Fax: 350 76293

3
SPAIN
(Member of the European Union)

GENERAL INFORMATION

CRUISING AREAS

The Mediterranean coast of Spain has several major traditional cities, such as Barcelona, Valencia and Alicante, together with a considerable number of tourist developments and marinas. The Balearic Islands form a delightful cruising ground. Many small fishing ports are available to pleasure craft.

Care should be taken with the security of a yacht left unattended in the larger ports.

Spanish yacht clubs tend to be very exclusive and expect high standards of dress and behaviour from their members. Visitors are likely to be welcome only if they respect this attitude.

The Cabrera Archipelago, south of Majorca, is a National Park and a permit (free) is required. Application should be made three weeks before required.
Tel: (971) 465507 (Palma de Mallorca)
Fax: (971) 465700

MAJOR HARBOURS AND MARINAS

The Spanish Tourist Office publish detailed maps listing marina and harbour facilities, instalaciones nauticas, covering the regions of Andalucia, Balearics, Catalonia. A number of marinas provide lifting-out facilities.

OTHER INFORMATION

The unit of currency is the peseta.
Tel. code from the UK: 00 34
Tel. code to the UK: 07 44

STD calls may be made to the UK from public call boxes which have instructions in English. 25 and 100 peseta coins are required. A 75% reduction applies after 2000.

ENTRY BY SEA

PORTS OF ENTRY

There are no specified ports of entry, but if arriving from a non-EU country the first entry must be made at a port large enough to include a Customs office.

CUSTOMS

EU regulations apply.

TARIF G5

Vessels are liable to be required to pay a fee known as Tarif G5, which can represent a significant surcharge on the normal cost of berthing. The tax described, as a Port Tax, varies from area to area but in the Valencia district is levied at 800 pesetas x length (m) x beam (m). (About £180 for a 10 m. vessel in 1997). Smaller marinas, not classified as ports, apparently do not make this charge.

DUTIABLE STORES

EU regulations apply.

ENTRY BY ROAD

EU Customs regulations apply.

TEMPORARY IMPORTATION

EU customs regulations apply.

Non-Spanish nationals living in Spain for more than six months in any one year are required to re-register their vessels on the Spanish register, thereby attracting a 12% registration tax and a requirement to comply with all Spanish licencing and equipment carriage regulations.

A UK national permanently resident in Spain loses the entitlement to the Small Ships Register but retains the right to UK Registration if the vessel is owned by a UK established person or company.

DOCUMENTATION

DOCUMENTATION OF VESSEL

Ship's registration papers, ship radio licence and evidence of marine insurance cover should be carried as should proof of VAT status.

DOCUMENTATION OF CREW

No certificates of competence are required on UK flagged vessels. However in a country where officials are used to seeing certificates an ICC is always useful. RYA certificates are accepted on Spanish flagged vessels.

Yachtmaster Ocean = Capitan de Yate
Yachtmaster Offshore = Patron de Yate (de altura)
Coastal Skipper = Patron de Yate
Day Skipper = Patron de embarcaciones de recreo.
ICC = Patron de embarcaciones de recreo restringido a motor.

RYA certificates can also be converted to their Spanish equivalent.

CHARTERING

There are numerous charter companies which operate in Spain and the Balearics. Advertisements will be found in the major yachting magazines.

FUEL, STORES AND REPAIRS

Diesel is available at most ports and Camping Gaz is universally available. It is not easy to get other sorts of gas cylinders filled. Paraffin is difficult to obtain but 'lamp oil' is available in some large supermarkets and DIY stores. There are good repair facilities in many of the marinas and local workshops. Spares and electronic equipment are available in the larger marinas. There are excellent markets for fish, fruit and vegetables. Water is readily available and is normally potable. Wine, beer and local spirits are cheap and plentiful. A *permiso aduarnero* form from Customs will enable stores to be imported duty free.

WEATHER FORECASTS

On the South Coast, forecasts from Gibraltar can be picked up. Further north and in the Balearics, the best source is Radio Marseille (see under France). Most yacht clubs and marinas post a daily forecast and synoptic chart, sometimes translated into English. Radio Monaco on SSB gives English language forecasts for the whole Western Mediterranean twice daily

PUBLICATIONS

British Admiralty charts are excellent for use in Spanish waters and the information is now largely obtained from Spanish charts. Spanish charts, fully updated, are published by Instituto Hydrografico de la Marina at Cadiz and are obtainable there, or at any Libreria Nautica.

Admiralty Sailing Directions
Mediterranean Pilot Vol 1
Mediterainean Spain, RRC Pilotage Foundation (Imray) 1998
Islas Baleares, RCC Pilotage Foundation (Imray) 1997
Imray M series charts, M1, M2 & M3.
Marina Guide – Mediterranean (Vetus).
In Spanish - Derroteros - which contains excellent pictures of the coast.
Instalaciones Nauticas (Spanish Tourist Office).

USEFUL ADDRESSES

Spanish Embassy, 24 Belgrave Square, London SW1 Tel: 0171 235 5555.

Spanish Consulate, 20 Draycott Place, London SW3 2RZ Tel: 0171 589 8989.

Spanish National Tourist Office,
57/58 St James's St., London SW1
Tel: 0171 499 0901.

Spanish Chamber of Commerce, 5 Cavendish Square, London W1 Tel: 0171 637 9061.

Direccion General de la Marina Mercante, Ruiz de Alarconi, 28014 Madrid.

Real Club Nautico de Barcelona, Tiglado 9, Barcelona.

Federacion Espanola de Vela, Juan Vigon 23, Madrid 3.

Real Automovil Club de Espana,
General Sanjurjo 10, Madrid 3.

Salon Nautico International, Avda. Reina Maria Christina, Palacio 1, Barcelona.

Liga Naval Espanola, Silva 6, Madrid.

Camper & Nicholsons (Spain) S.A.
Club de Mar, Palma de Mallorca, Spain.

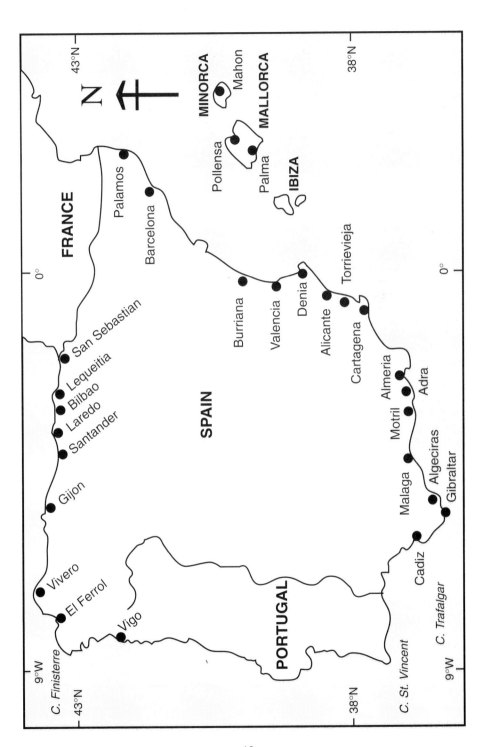

4
FRANCE AND CORSICA
(Member of the European Union)

GENERAL INFORMATION

CRUISING AREAS

The French Mediterranean coast stretches for 300M between the Spanish and Italian frontiers. In the west is the Languedoc-Roussillon region and the Camargue. There are numerous large new marinas.

The Cote Bleu runs from the Rhone to Toulon; there are small fishing harbours, marinas and the major port of Marseilles.

Further east is the very fashionable area of the Cote d'Azure and Riviera. There are many marinas, the facilities are excellent but they can be expensive and crowded. Cruising tends to be from one marina to another.

Corsica is one of the most beautiful islands in the Mediterranean with numerous anchorages and small harbours, as well as marinas at Porto Vecchio, Bonifacio and Calvi. Some anchorages can be crowded at the height of the season but it is possible to cruise in comfort at other times.

OTHER INFORMATION

The unit of currency is the French franc.

Tel. code from the UK: 00 33

Tel. code to the UK: 19 44

To contact a yacht from ashore in France the number to call is 19 39 00. The caller must state the name of the vessel, its call-sign and the name of the person required, also details of the area in which the yacht is cruising and the type of radio on board.

Clean mooring zones have been established in 10 selected bays between La Ciotat and Menton. Yachts are encouraged not to discharge sewage and this will eventually become mandatory.

ENTRY BY SEA

PORTS OF ENTRY

A list of ports of entry is not published; all major ports have Customs and Immigration offices.

CUSTOMS

EU regulations apply, but the French have been very slow in applying the VAT rules for EU residents. As a result VAT paid and VAT unpaid vessels, owned by EU residents, exist side by side.

However, on the Atlantic coast of France, non-EU visitors have been fined for spending more than 6 months in any 12 in the EU. Non-EU visitors should not visit France if they been in the EU for more than 6 months in the last 12 without first checking with French Customs. Once a non-French EU citizen has been in France continuously for 6 months, a boat tax, known as a Passport, is payable

DUTIABLE STORES

EU regulations apply.

ENTRY BY ROAD

EU Customs regulations apply.

There are no special rules applying to trailing or car-topping boats into France. Generally speaking, provided that you comply with the regulations for towing in the UK, you will have complied sufficiently with French trailing law.

If the overall length of vehicle and trailer (including the boat) exceeds 18m, or if the width is greater than 2.5m, you must seek police permission to travel as a large load.

TEMPORARY IMPORTATION

EU regulations apply.

DOCUMENTATION

DOCUMENTATION OF VESSEL

Ship's registration papers, the original, not a photocopy, must be on board at all times.

The only craft exempt from this rule are those small enough to be classified as *engin de plage* (beach toy), for a definition see Appendix A.

DOCUMENTATION OF CREW

EU regulations apply.

There is no requirement for a certificate of competence or the carriage of particular equipment for British flagged vessels cruising the French coast. However, anyone at the helm of a French flagged vessel, without a certificate of competence issued by their own government, will need either a *carte de mer* for craft powered by engines between 6hp and 50hp operating in daylight hours within five miles of a harbour, or a *permis mer* for craft outside these limits. A coastal version of the *permis mer* is available for craft powered by engines of more than 50hp and for use day or night but within five miles of the coast. These French certificates are not available outside France, but a foreigner carrying a certificate of competence issued on behalf of their own government may drive a French flagged leisure motorcraft covered by that certificate.

Note: The RYA is authorised by the UK Government to issue the ICC.

INLAND WATERWAYS

A Certificate of Competence ∙nd a copy of the CEVNI Rules, contained in the *RYA Book of EuroRegs*, must be carried.

A licence is required to navigate on the French canals. It is obtainable from the local VNF office, addresses from the French Government Tourist Office.

Full details of the routes from the English Channel to the Mediterranean are included in C1/98. Further information on the Rhone can be obtained from:

Service de la Navigation
2 Quai de la Quarantine
69321 Lyon Cedex 1
and on the Canal du Midi from:
Service de la Navigation
8 Port St Etienne
Tel: 61 80 07 18

More general information on the inland waterways can be requested from:

Secretary of State for Transport by Roads and Inland Waterways
L'Arche de la Defense (Pilier Sud)
92055 Paris la Defense
Tel: 40 81 21 22

The skippers of all vessels navigating French inland waters, which in general terms begin at the first obstacle to navigation for sea-going ships, need to hold a valid certificate of competence. Only persons over 16 may helm on French inland waters. On major rivers the start of inland waters is defined as -

Garonne, Pont de Pierre in Bordeaux;

Dordogne, Pont de Pierre in Libourne; Loire, Pont Handandine or Pont de Pirmil; Rhone, Pont de Trinquetaille in Arles; Seine, Pont Jeanne d'Arc in Rouen.

On smaller rivers the mouth, excluding the coastal town, is taken as the limit of inland water.

Category C licence - *coches de plaisance*. For those driving vessels less than 15 metres in length. A Certificate of Competence is accepted by the French as an alternative as long as a copy of the CEVNI rules is carried.

Category PP licence - *peniches de plaisance*. For those driving vessels longer than 15 metres. There is no equivalent available in the UK, the French government have not yet decided what UK certificate they will accept, in practice the ICC appears acceptable. Note, no certificate is needed for dinghies without motors or for other vessels less than 5 metres in length and not capable of exceeding 20kph.

The registered number of the vessel must be displayed on both sides in letters and figures 150mm high. The registration book must be carried on board whenever the vessel is moving.

The carriage of masts across France while vessels navigate the inland waters can be arranged by:

Navy Service, Ave de la 1st DFL,
13230 Port St.Louis du Rhone.
Tel: +442 11 0055 Fax: +442 48 4506 or by:
Chantier Naval, de la Baie de Seine,
136 Quai Frimard, 76600 Le Haure
Tel: +235 25 30 51
The cost is likely to be about £500 incl taxes.

FUEL, STORES AND REPAIRS

There is little problem in obtaining provisions of all kinds from shops, supermarkets and markets. Camping Gaz, diesel and water are readily available in all ports.

Red diesel is only available for use in generators or in central heating systems and must not be used for the boat's engines. However red diesel in the tanks when a vessel arrives in France may be used. It is wise to retain a receipt to prove purchase outside France. Red diesel imported in cans is liable to duty.

Many of the marinas have good repair and laying-up facilities. Spares can generally be obtained or shipped from the UK without too much difficulty.

You may find a small Italian tanker which sometimes positions itself in International waters at the French/Italian border and sells duty-free diesel.

NAVIGATIONAL AIDS

Buoyage, lights and RDF coverage are good both on the mainland and Corsica.

WEATHER FORECASTS

There are excellent forecasts (in French) which are easily understood as they are read at dictation speed. A tape recorder may be useful. Ch.23 and Nice Radio (106.3 and 106.5) give regular bulletins in English.

Principal stations are:

Marseilles 1906kHz; 2649 - 3792kHz
Monaco - 8728kHz.

Full details of French forecasts are available in a pamphlet issued by Météo France, available at most French Harbours and Marinas or direct from Météo France. 1 Quai Branly, 75340 Codex 07. Tel: 0145 56 71 71

A subscription service for faxed synoptic charts and area forecasts can be arringed by writing to Météo France at this address.

PUBLICATIONS

Admiralty Sailing Directions Vols I & II
South France Pilot (several volumes) *Brandon* (Imray)

Mediterranean France and Corsica - A Sea Guide *Heikell* (Imray)
CEVNI rules - The RYA Book of EuroRegs, available from the RYA

USEFUL ADDRESSES

French Consulate General, 21 Cromwell Road, London SW7 2DQ. Tel: 0171 838 2000.

French Government Tourist Office, 178 Piccadilly, London W1V 0AL Tel: 0891 244123

Touring Club de France, 178 Piccadilly, London W1V 0AL.

Touring Club de France, Service Nautique, 65 Avenue de la Grande Armee, 75782 Paris. Cedex 16 Tel: 502 1400.

Federation Francaise du Yachting a Voile, 55 Rue Kleber, Paris Tel: 4505 6800.

Centre de Renseignements Douanier, 8 Rue de la Tour des Dames, 75009 Paris Tel: 4260 3590.

Ministeres des Transports, Direction General des Transports Interieurs, Direction des Transport Terrestres (sous Direction des Voies Navigables), 244-246 Boulevard Saint Germain 75007, Paris.

Service Hydrographique et Oceanographique de la Marine
13 Rue du Chatelier, Epshom
BP 426, 29275 Brest Tel: 9803 0917

APPENDIX A

Definition of a Beach Toy *(Engin de Plage)*

The rule requiring registration of boats is relaxed for Beach Toys. These craft are not permitted to go more than 300m offshore.

They are defined as follows:

Rigid craft:

1. Rigid single-handed sailing craft and canoes:
   Beam less than 1.15m and Product of length x beam x depth less than 1.5m³.

2. Other rigid craft (sail or motor):
   Beam less than 1.2m and Product of length x beam x depth less than 2.0m³.

Dinghy sailors will find that the dividing line falls somewhere between a Laser (which

requires registration) and a Topper (which is exempt).

Inflatable craft:

1. Motorised inflatables:
   Length less than 2.75m and Beam less than 1.2m and Air Volume less than 350 litres

2. Sailing inflatables:
   Length less than 3.7m and Sail area less than 7m²

Other craft exempt from registration:

1. Windsurfers (Sailboards)

2. Aquabikes (Jet-skis)

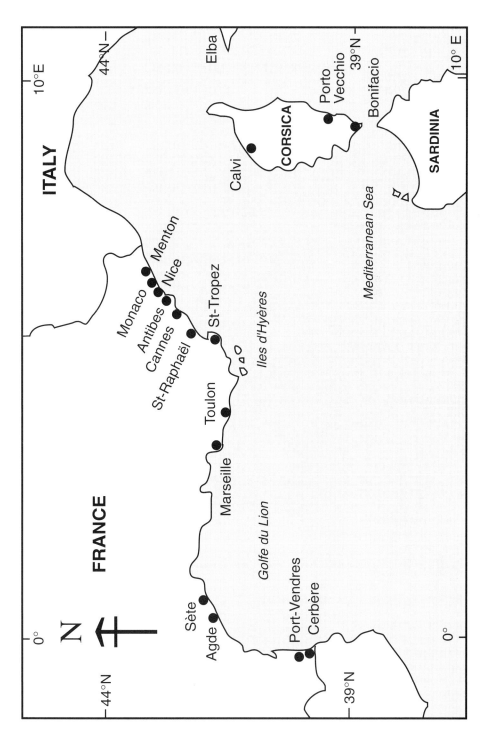

5
ITALY
(Member of the European Union).

GENERAL INFORMATION

CRUISING AREAS

The Italian Riviera from the French border to Tuscany is a beautiful coast with much to offer, including numerous well-equipped marinas. This popular area is crowded in the summer months.

The Tuscan coast and archipelago offer marinas, harbours and anchorages which will also be crowded in summer.

The Tyrrenhian seaboard of Italy is crowded in its northern part because of the proximity to Rome, and local yachts leave little space for the visitor. South of Naples the coast is less busy.

Sardinia is a beautiful cruising ground, uncrowded except in the North East in August. The east coast of Sardinia is rather exposed with limited safe shelter and should be navigated with due attention to the weather.

The northern part of Sicily is an interesting cruising area and gives access to the various islands in the southern part of the Tyrrenhian Sea. The southern coast of Sicily is not well known as a cruising area but contains some of the finest archeological sites outside Greece and Turkey.

From the toe to the boot of Italy is not popular for cruising but is useful for passage making to Greece and former Yugoslavia.

The east coast of Italy is not an attractive area for visiting yachts.

The north coast from Venice to Trieste has many marinas where both Italian and foreign yachts are kept.

Special rules apply on the Italian lakes. They are displayed in various languages at the lakeside. Documents must be carried on board.

PORTS AND MARINAS

There are many marinas, fishing ports and anchorages and the Italian Waters Pilot is the best source of information. Many marinas in the popular areas are very crowded in the season. Italian marinas can be very expensive.

OTHER INFORMATION

Banking hours are from 0830 to 1320 and for one hour in the afternoon – generally 1500 to 1600.

The unit of currency is the lira (ITL).

Tel. code from the UK: 00 39

Tel. code to the UK: 00 44

Italian callboxes use a special token called a gettone or 100 and 200 lira coins and pre-paid phone cards.

ENTRY BY SEA

PORTS OF ENTRY

There are no specific ports of entry; any major port will have Customs and Immigration facilities.

CUSTOMS

EU regulations apply.

ENTRY BY ROAD

No Customs papers are needed for boats with or without engines or when brought by car and trailer and having the same number plate. Boats must be inspected by a Port Authority before entering the water on some lakes.

Boats with engines require insurance with the third party clause translated into Italian.

TEMPORARY IMPORTATION

EU regulations apply.

DOCUMENTATION

DOCUMENTATION OF VESSEL

Ship's registration papers.

A certificate of insurance with an Italian translation; this may not always be asked for but is nonetheless essential. The regulation concerned states that a visiting foreign yacht must have 'a Certificate of Insurance for third party liabilities issued by an Insurance Company having reciprocal arrangements with a recognised Italian Insurance Company'. It is therefore advisable to check with one's insurance company that this recognition exists, when asking them to supply the translation.

Third party insurance complying with the regulation may be obtained in Italy quite cheaply through an insurance broker – the document is then, of course, in Italian.

Proof of VAT status should be carried. A crew list is useful, it should read: surname, fore name, date and place of birth, function on board, passport number and nationality.

RECREATIONAL CRAFT DIRECTIVE

Italian law links boat design categories to authorised areas of use. When published this was under review.

DOCUMENTATION OF CREW

EU regulations apply.

Foreigners carrying a certificate of competence from their own country may navigate the craft for which they are qualified. It is advisable to carry the International Certificate of Competence, particularly on motor cruisers.

CHARTERING

The Traveller's Handbook, which may be obtained from the Italian Tourist Board, contains a list of yacht charterers.

FUEL, STORES AND REPAIRS

Yacht repairs of all kinds are available in the major centres. Some marinas have lifting facilities. In smaller harbours help is usually available although it may be from a garage rather than a marine engineer.

Provisions are easily obtained from supermarkets and general stores. Diesel and water are available in most marinas and harbours, and Camping Gaz is readily available in shopping areas. Credit cards may not be accepted for fuel purchases.

You may find a small tanker which sometimes positions itself in International waters at the French/Italian border and sells duty-free diesel.

NAVIGATIONAL AIDS

There is good buoyage and lights as well as numerous radio beacons.

WEATHER FORECASTS

The national radio station (Radio Uno) broadcasts forecasts in Italian for the whole of the Mediterranean at around 0640, 1530 and 2235 on 658kHz, 1035kHz and 1575kHz. The forecasts are read slowly, and are easy to follow. Monaco radio on SSB

Ch.25, 26 and 27 at 0935, 1535 and 2135 local, give good forecasts in Italian followed by English. VHF Ch 68 - continuous service. This can be received throughout the whole west coast of Italy.

PUBLICATIONS

It is wise to obtain BA Charts of the areas one intends to visit before leaving the UK as this avoids possible linguistic and conventional sign problems, but Italian charts are easily readable and up to date. They can be obtained in large ports (eg Genoa and Naples) from the Italian Naval Authorities.

BA Charts and Pilot Books cover the whole area. Most yacht chandlers sell large scale plastic covered yachting charts but these are rather expensive.

The Tyrrenhian Sea *Denham* (John Murray). Admiralty Sailing Directions, Mediterranean Pilots Vols 1,2,3.

Travellers' Handbook (Italian State Tourist Office) – gratis.

Italian Waters Pilot *Heikell* (Imray) (1998).

Adriatic Pilot *Thompson* (Imray) supplement (1999).

Vade-Marino for National Tourism in Italy (Italian State Tourist Office).

USEFUL ADDRESSES

Italian Consulate General, 38 Eaton Place, London SW1 Tel: 0171 235 9371

ENIT – Italian State Tourist Office, 1 Princes Street, London W1R 8AY Tel: 0171 408 1254

Federazione Italiana Vela, V. Brigata, Bisagno 2, Genoa, Italy Tel: 39 010 56 50 83

Federazione Italiana Motonautica, Via Cappuccio, 19 Milano.

Federazione Italiana Sci Nautico (water skiing), Viale Rimembranze di Greco, 1 Milano.

Federazione Italiana Canottaggio (rowing), Viale Tiziano, 70 Roma.

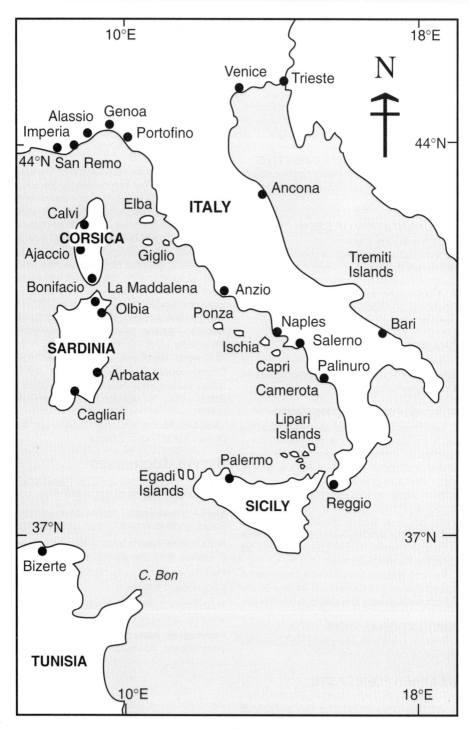

6
SLOVENIA - CROATIA - MONTENEGRO

GENERAL INFORMATION

CRUISING AREAS

The coastline of the former Yugoslavia, now divided into Slovenia, Serbia, Croatia, Bosnia Hercegovina and Montenegro, is one of Europe's most indented and beautiful coastlines, and close offshore there are over 700 islands. Almost everywhere the mountains come steeply to the sea; the scenery is magnificent and the water clear.

There is good cruising in the small section of coast which is now Slovenia, but it is Croatia which provides the most attractive environment for the cruising yachtsman. There is perhaps rather less hassle on this coast than before the war as the Yugoslavian Federal Forces have withdrawn and can no longer restrict access to places.

The major cruising areas are:
- the northern Adriatic Islands of the Kvarner Gulf;
- the Karnati Islands in the region of Zadar (although it is best to check on the local political situation before visiting mainland harbours or anchorages);
- the islands to the south of Split.

The coast and islands of Slovenia and Croatia have been open and freely visited by yachts since 1996. The coastline of Montenegro, which incudes the outstandingly beautiful Gulf of Kotor, is now open to cruising yachts.

ENTRY BY ROAD

British insurance companies are sometimes reluctant to provide green cards owing to their lack of up-to-date knowledge of the political situation. However, with perseverance it is possible to get the necessary documentation. The country code for the green card is HR (Hrvatska) for Croatia and SLO for Slovenia. Insurance agents are not always aware of this. Insurance is available at the borders.

SLOVENIA

Slovenia contains the well appointed marina at Portoros.

ENTRY BY SEA

Koper or Piran (all year), Izola (May to October only). Departure by sea must also be reported to the maritime authorities.

MINIMUM EQUIPMENT

Regardless of the country of registration all vessels used in Slovenian waters must carry: A suitable anchor with at least 30m of rope or chain. A mooring rope at least 10m long Two paddles. Bilge pump. First aid kit Six hand flares

CROATIA AND MONTENEGRO

MAJOR HARBOURS AND MARINAS

The Adriatic Croatia International Club (ACI) operates a large number of marinas along this coast and is still expanding. In addition there are a number of independent marinas such as Marina Veruda near Pula.

There are many beautiful and secure anchorages amongst the islands although in the high season insects can be a problem. National park areas make a small charge for anchoring, but the areas are kept clean and free from wasps, flies and mosquitoes.

It is reported that a yacht cruised the Gulf of Kotor in 1997 and apart from frequent military checks were not unduly hindered apart from when they re-entered Croatian waters.

In view of the current situation in Kosovo caution should be exercised when visiting the area. Advice should be sought from the Foreign and Commonwealth Office.

OTHER INFORMATION

The official currency is the kuna, which is pegged to the German mark. In practice this means that the exchange rate is normally in the region of 8.8 kuna to £1 (December 1996).

A tourist tax of about 2DM per day per person is collected by marinas along with the berthing charge, which is normally around 30-40DM per day (January 1995). Annual contract holders in their home marinas pay a consolidated fee of 50 DM annually (excluding

marina charges).
Tel. code from the UK: 00 385
Tel. code to the UK from Croatia: 99 44

ENTRY BY SEA

CUSTOMS

Customs clearance must be obtained on arrival from a foreign country. Officials are normally very helpful and courteous.

DUTIABLE STORES

The main preoccupation is with drugs and firearms rather than alcoholic beverages, unless excessive quantities are being carried.

DOCUMENTATION

DOCUMENTATION OF VESSEL

Ship's registration papers.

A cruising permit must be obtained on arrival. Cruising permits are only issued for 12 months from date of issue. For boats 12-15 metres the cost is about £140. A crew list must be attached to the cruising permit and updated in line with any crew change. In Croatia third party insurance must be carried. Vessels larger than 3 metres and jet skis must register with the harbour master.

DOCUMENTATION OF CREW

Passports are required.
Visas are not required.
Certificates of Competence are essential.
Crew list.

FUEL, STORES AND REPAIRS

Petrol and diesel are easily available. Expect to pay around 35p per litre for diesel.

Few spares are available locally but they can be imported duty free without difficulty.

CHARTERING

ACI Charter, M. Tita 221,51410, Opatija, Croatia. Tel: 010 385 51 271 1288 or 51 272570 or 213,4,5,6.

Fax 010 385 51 271824 or 51 712824

SAS Yachtcharter NTC Zlatna Croatia
Tel: 010 385 57 393 582 731
Fax: 010 385 57 393 588
In Slovenia it is illegal to charter from unregistered companies. Flotilla sailing was unavailable at the time of going to press

WEATHER FORECASTS

Available on VHF from Split, Zadar and Rijeka coast stations. From May 1 to October 1 continuous weather forecasts aimed at leisure craft and updated at 0700,1300 and 1900 are transmitted; first in Croat, then English, Italian and German. Ch.73 covers West Istrian Islands, Ch. 67 central coast and islands (Kornati islands to Vis), Ch. 73 SE coast and islands (Dubrovnik, Peljasic).

Italian national radio (Radio Uno) broadcasts forecasts in Italian for the whole Mediterranean and Adriatic on 1575kHz, 1035kHz and 658kHz at around 0640, 1530 and 2235. They are read slowly and are easy to understand.

PUBLICATIONS

The Croatian Hydrographic Office in Split publishes two excellent sets of 1:100,000 charts covering the entire coastline from Monfalcone in Italy to Ulcinj in Montenegro.

Admiralty Sailing Directions

Mediterranean Pilot Volume III (NP 47)

The Adriatic *Denham* (John Murray). Many former Yugoslav ports and anchorages are described.

The Adriatic Pilot *Thompson* (Imray 1990) with supplement (May 1999). The original is excellent and the supplement updates marina plans and includes extra anchorages and a very useful new passage.

The Adriatic Croatian Coast (Imray 1993).

The Yugoslav Coast, Guidebook and Atlas (Yugoslav Lexicographical Institute) obtainable from good bookshops in former Yugoslavia. A straightforward guidebook with good maps, packed with factual information.

USEFUL ADDRESSES

ACI Club, M. Tita 221, 51410 Opatija, Croatia Tel: 00 385 51 271288.
Fax: 00 385 51 271824.

Embassy of the Republic of Croatia, 18-21 Jermyn Street, London SW1Y 6HP Tel: 0171 434 2946 Fax: 0171 434 2953.

Embassy of Slovenia, 11-15 Wigmore Street, London W1 9LA Tel: 0171 495 7775.
Fax: 0171 287 7133.

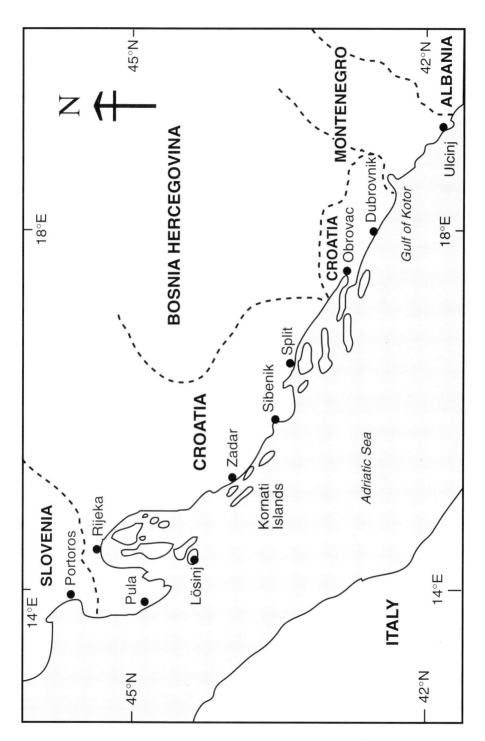

7
ALBANIA

GENERAL INFORMATION

We advise checking with the Foreign and Commonwealth Office for the latest advice before arrival in the country.

Visas for EU passport holders are free but US$5 entry tax is levied.

Detailed regulations for Albania are not known but it is advisable to carry yacht registration, certificate of competence and third party insurance.

A new marina is under construction.

Credit cards and travellers cheques are not accepted except on a limited basis in Terania. Yachts up to 30 tons are charged US$15 for their first visit then US$1 per metre per day depending on length of quayside occupied - moor stern to.

PORTS OF ENTRY

Durres
Vlore
Saranda
Shengjin

Entry procedure. 48 hours notice of arrival should be given on VHF Ch.15. Unannounced arrival can lead to a heavy fine or even seizure of the vessel. Vessels must report arrival to customs within 48 hours with a manifest (crew list), passports and visas, and health clearance from previous country. Vessels must notify harbour masters of next port of call for notification purposes and departure schedule for customs clearance.

8
MALTA

GENERAL INFORMATION

Malta is a convenient staging point for yachtsmen on passage in the central Mediterranean area. It has well-developed facilities for yachts and easy communications. English is widely spoken.

Malta is also an interesting cruising ground in its own right with picturesque harbours and attractive anchorages.

Owing to its geographical position at the centre of the trading routes of the Mediterranean, Malta has been an island of great strategic importance over the centuries and its history is both colourful and fascinating.

MAJOR HARBOURS AND MARINAS

The principal yachting port is Marsamxett Harbour with extensive yacht berths in Lazaretto Creek and Msida Creek. There is a small marina at Mgarr on the island of Gozo.

There are interesting harbours at Marsaxlokk in the south of the island, and at Mgarr.

Wintering facilities are available on the hard at Manoel Island. Marinas and hard standing can be very busy and advance booking is recommended.

Manoel Island – Telephone 330975

Msida Marina – Telephone 235713

Note that not all the harbours provide absolutely ideal shelter from all winds.

The presence on board of animals will preclude berthing alongside at any time. There are strict quarantine regulations.

OTHER INFORMATION

Tel. code from the UK: 00 356 (no area code is required in Malta)

Tel. code to the UK: 00 44

The unit of currency is the Maltese lira (MTL).

Maltese regulations are strictly enforced and should be closely adhered to.

ENTRY BY SEA

Yachts arriving from abroad should contact Malta Radio (Valletta) by VHF when within range for entry instructions. Normally clearance is in Msida Marina, but outside normal office hours a yacht may be asked to clear in Grand Harbour.

Before departure from Malta, a crew list and passports must be submitted to the Customs and Immigration officials.

PORTS OF ENTRY

Entry is normally made at Valletta, but in the summer months clearance in and out can be achieved at Mgarr on Gozo.

DUTIABLE STORES

Duty-free stores and fuel can be obtained by making arrangements with one of several agencies for completion of the necessary forms. 24 hours notice is required for fuel and up to 48 hours should be allowed for stores which will be delivered under Customs supervision. Customs require yachts to leave within 24 hours of embarking duty-free stores which may not be consumed within territorial waters.

DOCUMENTATION

DOCUMENTATION OF VESSEL

Ship's registration papers, Ship Radio Licence, a crew list in duplicate showing surname, forenames, passport numbers, nationality, status on board (i.e. crew member) and date of birth.

DOCUMENTATION OF CREW

Valid passports. It is necessary to obtain immigration cards from Immigration for each person on board to complete and sign. Crew members wishing to leave the yacht and return by air must report to the Port Police and have their passports stamped BEFORE going to the airport. There are no restrictions on crew changes.

CHARTERING

Details can be obtained from the Valletta Yacht Club (Telephone 331131). Charterers also advertise in UK yachting magazines.

FUEL, STORES AND REPAIRS

Good facilities exist at Manoel Island. Spares are not normally difficult to obtain.

General stores, wine and beer are available. Diesel, water and Camping Gaz are easily obtained. A van visits the quays with fresh vegetables and other supplies, however it is worthwhile remembering that the rate of exchange is £2 = £1 Maltese.

Water is metered. Misunderstandings have arisen in Lazaretto Creek with regard to water supply and close attention to the fittings and the meter reading, before and after water supply is recommended.

Fuel is available from an anchored barge in Valletta harbour.

NAVIGATIONAL AIDS

RDF beacons at Malta and Gozo.

WEATHER FORECASTS

Malta Radio transmits daily weather forecasts in English at 0803, 1203, 1803 and 2303 local time on 2625kHz and VHF 04 after preliminary calls on VHF 12.

PUBLICATIONS

BA Chart 194 covers Malta and there are also harbour charts.

Admiralty Sailing Directions
Mediterranean Pilot Vol 1
Ports and Anchorages Handbook
(Royal Malta YC)
The Yachtsman's Handbook and Cruising Guide to Malta (S & D Yachts) – gratis
Italian Waters Pilot *Heikell* (Imray)
North African Pilot *RCC* (Imray)

USEFUL ADDRESSES

Maltese High Commission, 36 Picadilly, London W1 Tel: 0171 292 4800.

Maltese Tourist Board, Malta House, 36-38 Picadilly, London W1 Tel: 0171 292 4900.

Thos. C Smith (Admiralty Chart Agents), 12 St. Christopher Street, Valletta.

S & D Yachts Ltd, 57 Gzira Road, Gzira, Malta Tel: 339908, 332259.

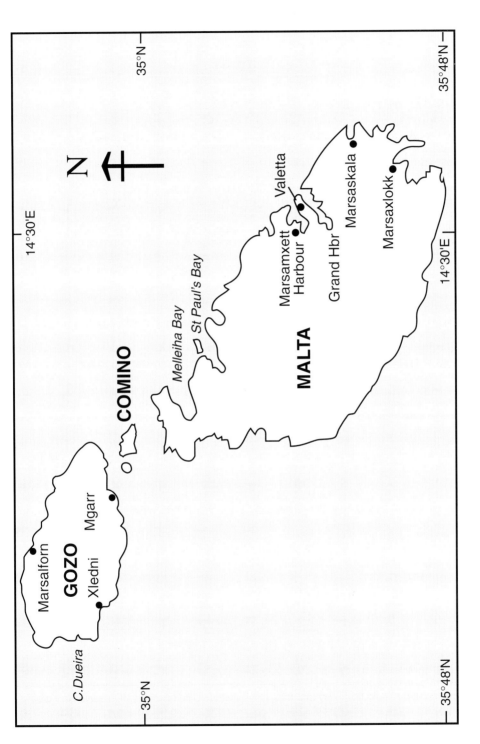

9
GREECE
(Member of the European Union)

GENERAL INFORMATION

Greece offers the yachtsman a great variety of picturesque places from which to choose – Aegean or Ionian Seas, remote or cosmopolitan islands, rocky or pine fringed beaches, quiet anchorages or sophisticated marinas. Everywhere are splendid reminders of the classical past from the site of the first naval engagement at Salamis to the cruising grounds of Ulysses. Supplies and provisions are readily available except on the more remote islands. Water can be in short supply on some islands.

CRUISING AREAS

The Ionian Sea, extending from Corfu to Zakynthos (about 140 miles) together with the Gulfs of Patras and Corinth (about 100 miles).

The Saronic and Argolic Gulfs, extending from the eastern end of the Corinth Canal to the south eastern coast of the Peloponnese (about 120 miles).

The Cyclades, the large group of 21 main islands in the central Aegean (about 120 miles W/E and 120 miles N/S).

Evia and the Northern Sporades, which include Skiathos and Skopelos.

The Northern Aegean, including Limnos, Lesvos, Khios and Samos - (about 150 miles N to S).

The Dodecanese, the Twelve Islands (actually 14) on the eastern side of the Aegean, stretching from Patmos in the north to Rhodes in the south (about 100 miles N/S).

Crete, and the Southern Peloponnese, including Kithera (about 250 miles from Zakynthos to Heraklion).

MAJOR HARBOURS AND MARINAS

There are hundreds of harbours and anchorages from which to choose. Most harbours are small fishing ports and not suitable for leaving a yacht unattended. The Greek National tourist organisation lists the following marinas but it should be noted that they are frequently very crowded and not necessarily suitable for leaving a yacht unattended.

Alimnos (Athens)	1000 berths	– Travel lift
Aretsou (Thesaloniki)	242 berths	– Travel lift
Flisvos (Athens)	375 berths	
Glifada (Athens)	780 berths	– Travel lift
Gouvia (Corfu)	480 berths	
Mandraki (Rhodes)	115 berths	
Methana (Saronic)	70 berths	
Olympic Marina	50 berths	
Patras	400 berths	
Porto Carras (Khalkidikli)	170 berths	
Vouliagmeni (Athens)	115 berths	
Zea (Athens)	950 berths	

It is still possible to find creeks and coves with good shelter, room to swing, fine scenery and not another yacht or house in sight. In harbour it is customary to berth bow or stern to quay wherever there is room and to avoid the berth used by the inter-island ferries. Blue and yellow diagonal stripes painted on a portion of the quay indicate the refuelling point for yachts. This berth must be left free if you are not refuelling.

Berth charges which vary according to the length of stay and yacht size are payable in all Greek marinas. In some these charges are based on the Gross Registered Tonnage (GRT). These charges include the use of the berth and harbour facilities but separate fees are charged for water, electricity, telephone and other services. At many ports you will be asked by the Harbour Police to visit their office with your papers. You are then asked to pay the berthing fee. Charges are levied in all harbours and sometimes when at anchor.

The power supply in Greece is 50Hz – 220V.

There are a number of marinas and yacht harbours on the coasts of Attica near Greater Athens. These are often very crowded in the summer months.

Greek authorities have levied fines for yachts flying torn or worn Greek courtesy flags and for dinghies not carrying safety equipment. This includes lifejackets and flares even in a rubber dinghy setting out on a swimming trip.

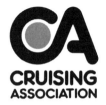

Join now . . .
Make friends with the
Cruising Association

CRUISING
ASSOCIATION

What does the CA offer you?

- UK and worldwide network of local representatives

- Representation for the cruising yachtsmen and women at national and local level

- A new purpose built, headquarters in London with every possible facility

- Local Sections in many parts of the country offering a range of activities

- A wide variety of publications for the cruising yachtsman

- Winter lectures and events including RYA theory and other courses

- Crewing Service to put skippers in touch with crew and crew with skippers

**Complete the form overleaf
or telephone 0171 537 2828**

APPLICATION FOR MEMBERSHIP

Surname _____

Forename _____

Initials _____

Decorations _____

Address _____

_____

_____

Post Code _____

I give my permission to publish my address in the CA Yearbook

Home Tel. _____ Fax. _____

Work Tel. _____ Fax. _____

Mobile _____

Do you belong to any Yacht Clubs or associations? If yes please list

_____

_____

Boat Name _____

Class _____

Rig _____

LOA _____

Home Port _____

I hereby apply to become a member of the Cruising Association and agree, if elected by the council, to abide by the rules, regulations and code of the Association.

I enclose £ _____ as payment for this year's subscription and the Direct Debit Mandate for future years.

Signed _____

MEMBERSHIP RATES 1999

	Entrance Fee	Annual Subscription Cash	Annual Subscription Direct Debit		Annual Subscription Cash	Annual Subscription Direct Debit
Ordinary Member	£10*	£91	£85	Young Member (under 25)	£23	£20
Spouse Ordinary Member		£26	£23			
				Cadet Member (under 18)	£10	–
Overseas Member	£10*	£44	–			
Spouse Overseas Member		£17	–			

* Members of The Royal Cruising Club, The Irish Cruising Club, The Clyde Cruising Club, plus holders of The Royal Yachting Association Yachtmaster Offshore Certificate (both theory and practical) are not required to pay an entrance fee.

DIRECT DEBIT MANDATE

National Westminster Bank plc, Mincing Lane Branch, Fenchurch Street, London EC3M 3JH

The Association undertakes not to debit any amount other than annual subscriptions

To the Manager (your Bank)

Bank _____ plc

Branch _____

Address _____

_____

_____

Post Code _____

I/We authorise you until further notice in writing to charge my/our account on or immediately after the anniversary of joining date unspecified amounts which the Cruising Association may originate by Direct Debit.

Full Name of account to be debited

_____

Bank Account No.

_____

Sort Code

_____

Signed _____

PRINT Name _____

Date _____

Banks may decline to accept instructions for direct debits to other than current accounts.

When completed please detach and return to:

CA
CRUISING ASSOCIATION

The Cruising Association
CA House, 1 Northey Street
Limehouse Basin, London E14 8BT
Tel: 0171 537 2828 Fax: 0171 537 2266

Join the RYA...

Personal membership costs very little . . . and means a <u>great deal</u>

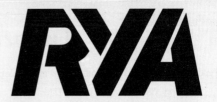

Why join?

Being a member of the RYA means that you can:

- use the expert legal, cruising, racing and windsurfing advice services when you need them

- obtain up to date information on training, moorings, navigation and foreign cruising procedures

- help the RYA protect its members' activities from outside interference and unnecessary bureaucracy

- make use of the special RYA restaurant and lounge at selected boat shows

- benefit from the free offers and discounts available

What free offers are available to RYA members?

- The International Certificate of Competence (useful for those who cruise abroad)

- Allocation of a sail number

- Two RYA publications a year, (choose from a whole range of subjects), a book token worth £5.00 (on selected publishers books from the RYA catalogue) or an RYA diary

- Quarterly magazine delivered to your home

- RYA Visa Card - no annual fee (application subject to status)

Windsurfing members receive third party insurance and one RYA publication or a book token worth £2.50.

Junior members receive one free RYA publication and a windsurfing junior member receives the third party insurance only.

How about discounts?

- 10% (or more depending on qualifications) reduction on yacht insurance arranged through the RYA Brokers Bishop Skinner and Co. Ltd.

- Reduction on measurement certificate fees

Will my membership make a difference?

Yes. With every new member the RYA strengthens its voice to speak up and represent the interests of individuals - people like you who go afloat in their spare time. Not everyone views boating in quite the same way as RYA members. Pressure from other organisations such as the EU, port authorities, the environmental lobby and the foreshore landowners can affect your freedom afloat.

YOUR MEMBERSHIP MATTERS

How can I make my voice heard?

Write to the RYA expressing your opinions and attend the AGM. It is a democratic organisation and your views are important.

How much does it cost?

An adult personal member (£23 by direct debit)	£25
A family membership (£38 by direct debit).	£40
Under 21	£10

Please fill in the membership form overleaf

RYA MEMBERSHIP Matters

Yes I want to join the RYA

Type of Membership Required: (tick as applicable)

☐ **Personal £25** (*£23* if you pay by Direct Debit)

☐ **Family £40** (*£38* if you pay by Direct Debit)

☐ **Under 21 £10**

Please indicate your main boating interest by ticking one box only	W	SC	SR	PR	MC	PW
	☐	☐	☐	☐	☐	☐

W=Windsurfing   SC=Sail Cruising
SR=Sail Racing   PR=Powerboat Racing
MC=Motor Cruising   PW=Personal Watercraft

	Title	Forename	Surname	Date of Birth	Male	Female
1.						
2.						
3.						
4.						

Address

Town   County   Postcode

Signature _____

RYA

Instructions to your Bank or Building Society to pay by Direct Debit

DIRECT Debit

Please complete this form and return it to: **Royal Yachting Association**, RYA House, Romsey Road, Eastleigh, Hampshire SO50 9YA.

To The Manager: **Bank/Building Society**

Address:

Post Code:

Originators Identification Number

9	5	5	2	1	3

5. RYA Membership Number (For office use only)

2. Name(s) of account holder(s)

3. Branch Sort Code

☐☐ — ☐☐ — ☐☐

4. Bank or Building Society account number

☐☐ . ☐☐☐☐☐

6. Instruction to pay your Bank or Building Society
Please pay Royal Yachting Association Direct Debits from the account detailed in this instruction subject to the safeguards assured by The Direct Debit Guarantee.
I understand that this instruction may remain with the Royal Yachting Association and, if so, details will be passed electronically to my Bank/Building Society.

Signature(s) _____

Date _____

Banks and Building Societies may not accept Direct Debit Instructions for some types of account

---

Cash, Cheque, Postal Order enclosed £ _____   Made payable to the Royal Yachting Association

077

Office use only: Membership No. Allocated

Office use / Centre Stamp

INLAND WATERWAYS

There are three waterways in Greece where special rules of navigation are in force.

The Corinth Canal. Designed to reduce the length of the voyage from Italian ports to Piraeus and the Eastern Mediterranean, this ship canal, 4M long and with a depth of 8 metres was opened for traffic in 1893. The canal authority is the state-owned Corinth Canal S.A.

As ships may not pass each other in the canal, permission to proceed must first be obtained by VHF Ch.11 from the canal authority at either end. Canal dues are paid at the eastern end. At all times comply with the flag and light signals which are clearly displayed at each end of the canal.

Corinth Canal dues are divided into categories depending on the size and purpose of the vessel. Yachts carrying fewer than 25 passengers are in category ST, and are calculated on Net Registered Tonnage. Yachts with SSR registration will be charged by length rather than GRT. There is a fixed charge plus a charge related to the yacht's length.

Pilotage is not compulsory for vessels under 800 tons. Normally, all craft in this category proceed under their own power, but tugs are available. In 1997 the charge for a 12m yacht, one way, was Dra 33,217.

The Evripos Channel. These narrows, which separate the Island of Euboea from the mainland, are crossed at Halkis by a sliding bridge. At times, a current of up to 8 knots flows through the narrows so that the bridge is only opened for shipping when tidal and weather conditions are favourable. This is normally at slack water and the bridge is only opened in the middle of the night to avoid disruption to road traffic. In 1997 the charge for a vessel up to 50 tonnes was Dra 2,000 plus 25% night supplement and 75% Sunday supplement plus VAT at 18% on total charge.

The Lefkas Canal. A canal separating the Island of Lefkas from the mainland has existed since classical times but the present ship canal and the long, northern breakwater were completed in the last century. Some 3M long and dredged to a minimum of 6 metres this provides a useful shortcut. At the northern end there is an opening bridge, the west end opens every hour on demand for yachts.

Currently north-going traffic goes first. Do not tow in the canal without prior permission. Towing of dinghies is accepted.

OTHER INFORMATION

It should be noted that serious legal implications could arise if a boat is used by a person other than the owner. The Greek authorities consider this to be chartering, and therefore illegal unless under a Greek flag. They are unwilling to accept a letter of authority as proof that a vessel is not under charter. This attitude is thought to be illegal within the EU but complaints to the Greek authorities by the RYA have produced no satisfactory answer. If a loan between friends is contemplated it is advisable to re-register the vessel, on the SSR, in the name or joint name of the proposed user.

It is apparently illegal for a non-Greek vessel to tow another vessel within the jurisdiction of a harbour.

Scuba diving is prohibited in most Greek waters, but is allowed in certain areas provided that detector instruments are not used and fishing is not undertaken. Local enquiries should be made.

All yachts should have holding tanks or biological treatment plants. Tanks may not be discharged closer than 6M from the nearest coast. Great care should be exercised when taking diesel on board to avoid spillage. Sea toilets should not be used in harbours. A small spillage of any kind will be very obvious and could result in a substantial and instant fine.

Tel. code from the UK: 00 30

Tel. code to the UK: 00 44

The unit of currency is the Greek drachma (GRD).

ENTRY BY SEA

EU regulations apply.

PORTS OF ENTRY

The listing of Ports of Entry is controversial. The official list, as published by the Greek National tourist organisation in 'Sailing the Greek Seas' seems to include ports which certainly do not have facilities for clearing in foreign yachts. The list which follows is not complete or official, but it is believed to include ports familiar with handling foreign yachts.

West coast:
Argostoli (Cephalonia – Ionian)
Katakolon (Peloponnese)
Kerkyra/Corfu (Corfu – Ionian)
Levkas (Ionian)
Patras (Gulf of Patras)
Preveza (Ionian)
Pylos (W Peloponnese)
Vathi (Ithaca – Ionian)
Zakynthos/Zante (Ionian)

Elsewhere:
Ayios Nikolaos (Crete)
Alexandroupolis (N Greece)
Chania (Crete)
Corinth (Gulf of Corinth)
Ermoupolis (Syros)
Iraklion (Crete)
Itea (Gulf of Corinth)
Kalamata (Peloponnese)
Kavala (N Greece)
Khios (Khios)
Kos (Kos)
Lavrion (Saronic Gulf)
Mirina (Limnos)
Mililini (Lesvos)
Navplion (Argolic Gulf)
Pithagorion (Samos)
Rhodes (Rhodes)
Thessaloniki (N Greece)
Volos (N Greece)
Vougliagmeni Marina (Saronic)
Zea Marina (Saronic)

CUSTOMS
EU regulations apply.

Note that Customs continue to be interested in whether a vessel is carrying drugs, firearms or scuba diving equipment, the latter because diving is forbidden in certain areas.

DUTIABLE STORES
EU regulations apply.

ENTRY BY ROAD
The normal passport regulations for visitors entering, staying in or leaving Greece also apply to those accompanying a boat and trailer. The width of the boat must not exceed 2.5m otherwise a special police permit may be required; the overall height of the boat on the trailer is restricted to 4m and the maximum combined length of the towing vehicle and the boat on the trailer is 15m. The speed limit on Greek toll roads is 100kph (62mph); 80kph is the rule on other roads, and in towns it is 50kph unless otherwise indicated on road signs. These limits also apply to cars towing a boat on a trailer or with a boat on the roofrack. Commercial vehicles carrying a boat are subject to the speed limits in force for the particular class of vehicle.

Pleasure craft (any small motor, sail or rowing boat) owned by non-EU residents whether on a trailer or roofrack will be permitted to enter Greece duty-free for 4 months – extendable on application to Customs. The boat will be entered on the owner's passport at the frontier and the owner will not be permitted to leave the country without the boat unless special arrangements are made with Customs.

In June 1996 the following list of crossing points with 24 hour Customs Offices was published by The Automobile and Touring Club of Greece.

Doirani, Euzoni, Niki, Promahonas, Ormenio, Kakavia, Kastanies, Kipi.

DOCUMENTATION

DOCUMENTATION OF VESSEL
Ship's registration papers. The Small Ships Register does not include reference to tonnage nor can it be adapted or modified to do so. Therefore, if higher charges are to be avoided, Part 1 Registration stating net tonnage is required for the Corinth Canal.

Vessels from other EU countries no longer need a transit log. EU vessels cannot buy duty free fuel. Transit logs are needed by non-EU vessels and these entitle the holder to purchase duty free fuel.

DOCUMENTATION OF CREW
Valid passports.

Greek regulations state 'A skipper's licence or other documentation of nautical qualifications and experience are required for pleasure boats under the Greek flag according to the size and type of vessel. For instance a speedboat licence is required for small fast-going vessels and for larger vessels reaching speeds above 25 knots, irrespective of other professional seamanship qualifications. Skippers of yachts under foreign flag should hold equivalent qualifications, issued by their home authorities or nautical clubs'.

International Certificate of Competence must be held. It should cover the type of vessel concerned.

CHARTERING

Cruising in Greek waters has become so popular in the last 10-15 years that chartering has developed from a small-scale occupation to an industry, which now offers over 2,000 craft to the cruising yachtsman. Many are based in the Athens-Piraeus area, but there are some sailing from Rhodes, Corfu, Thessaloniki and some other islands in the Aegean and Ionian Seas.

FUEL, STORES AND REPAIRS

Away from Athens spares are difficult to obtain and a yacht should be self-sufficient. Repairs to diesel engines are usually possible if the necessary spares are on board.

Diesel is readily available, as is Camping Gaz. Water is usually available but may be in short supply in the islands, which often have to rely on tanker delivery in the summer.

General provisions including meat, fish, vegetables and fruit are usually available at about the same price as in the UK.

NAVIGATIONAL AIDS

Except in major shipping areas, there is little buoyage. Lights are sparse and often low powered. Cruising in this area requires careful perusal of charts and pilots since hazards are not necessarily marked. It should be noted that local datum must be used for GPS or large errors will be encountered. In many cases Greek spelling or Greek script of place names and navigation aids leads to confusion when referring to non-Greek publications.

WEATHER FORECASTS

There are three sources of weather forecasts. The national radio broadcasts at 0630, first in Greek and then in English from Athens (729kHz) and Rhodes (1494kHz).

There is good Navtex reception from Corfu (K), Crete (H) and Limnos (L). Navtex reception is best from Crete (H). Greek TV broadcast a weather chart at 2130 . HF/SSB broadcast four times daily.

PUBLICATIONS

British Admiralty charts cover all the coasts and islands.

Greek charts are available from the Hellenic Navy Hydrographic Service.

Mediterranean Pilot Vol III (NP47) Ionian Sea and Gulf of Corinth.

Mediterranean Pilot Vol IV (NP48) Aegean Sea.

Ionian *Heikell* (Imray) 1996.

The Ionian Islands to the Anatolian Coast *Denham* (John Murray).

The Aegean *Denham* (John Murray).

The Greek Waters Pilot *Heikell* (Imray) 7th ed 1998

The Blue Guide – Greece (A & C Black).

Sailing the Greek Seas – from the Greek National Tourist Office.

USEFUL ADDRESSES

Greek Embassy 1A Holland Park, London W11 3JP Tel: 0171 221 6467.

Maritime Affairs Section - Embassy of Greece Maritime Consular.
Tel: 0171 727 0326. Fax: 0171 727 0509.

Greek National Tourist Organisation
4 Conduit Street, London W1R 0DJ
Tel: 0171 734 5997.

Automobile and Touring Club of Greece (ELPA), 2/4 Messogion, Athens 115 27
Tel: 748 8800. Fax: 778 6642.

British Embassy, Consular Department, Plutarchou Street, Athens 106 75.
Tel: Athens 7236 211.

British Admiralty Chart Agents,
85 Akti Miaouli,185 38, Piraeus
Tel: 4291181

New Company of Corinth Canal, Ithmia
Tel: 0741 37700.

Hellenic Navy Hydrographic Service,
Admiralty Building, Klafthmonos Square,
2, Paparrigopoulou St, Athens
Tel: Athens 32 0781, ext. 144 & 329 .

Port Police Directorate (for entry by sea)

Maritime and Tourism Section,
150 Gr. Labraki Street, 18518 Piraeus,
Tel: 4121211/4224784.
Fax: 4178101.

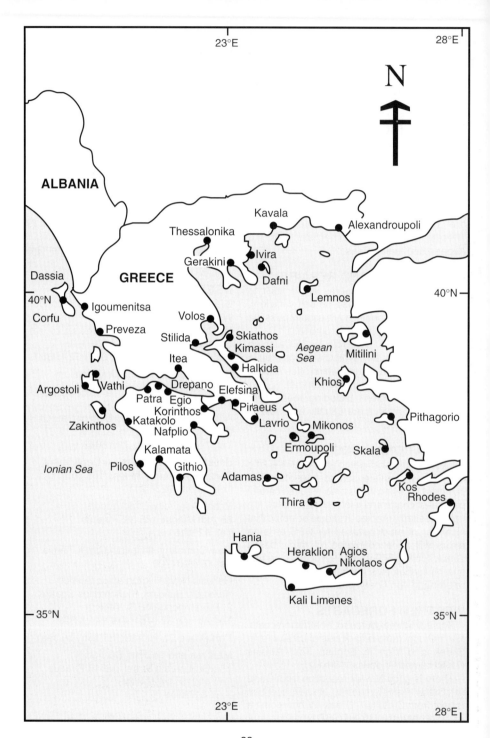

23°E
28°E

N

ALBANIA

Kavala

Thessalonika

Alexandroupoli

Gerakini

Ivira

Dassia

GREECE

Dafni

40°N

40°N

Corfu

Igoumenitsa

Lemnos

Preveza

Volos

Stilida

Skiathos

Kimassi

Aegean
Sea

Mitilini

Itea

Argostoli

Vathi

Drepano

Elefsina

Halkida

Khios

Patra

Egio

Korinthos

Piraeus

Pithagorio

Zakinthos

Katakolo

Nafplio

Lavrio

Mikonos

Kalamata

Ermoupoli

Skala

Ionian Sea

Pilos

Githio

Adamas

Kos

Thira

Rhodes

Hania

Heraklion

Agios
Nikolaos

Kali Limenes

35°N

35°N

23°E

28°E

10
CYPRUS

GENERAL INFORMATION

Cyprus is the third largest island in the Mediterranean and enjoys a mild climate with an average 340 days of bright sunshine each year. Summer winds are steady and, in winter, it is unusual for the sea and air temperatures to drop below 16°C and 9°C respectively.

Medical services and supplies are excellent.

Since July 1974 Cyprus has been divided by the Green Line patrolled by the UN. The northern sector is controlled by Turkey and is known as the Turkish Federated State of Northern Cyprus. It is not formally recognised by any country except Turkey. The southern sector, originally Greek controlled, is known as the Republic of Cyprus and is universally recognised. The Republic of Cyprus will not allow yachts which have called anywhere in Turkish held territory to enter any Republic harbour. They hold a blacklist of yachts.

Yachts may, however, proceed directly to and from the Republic of Cyprus and mainland Turkey.

NORTHERN CYPRUS

Northern Cyprus has fewer tourist facilities and is relatively unspoilt compared with the Republic of Cyprus.

The Greek language names which appear on charts and maps have been changed to Turkish names. Thus, for example, Nicosia is now Lefkoshia, Famagusta is Gazi Magusa and Kyrenia is Girne.

Gazi Magusa is the main commercial port of the north, but mooring facilities for yachts are poor; there are slipways but little else.

The small town of Girne on the north coast is 15M from Nicosia and only 45M from Turkey. It is a holiday resort with a small picturesque harbour. Entry fees are very reasonable but there is limited room for visiting yachts. There are no repair facilities and no chandlery. Diesel can be delivered to the quayside from a filling station about 200m from the harbour.

Yachts entering Northern Cyprus are required to fly the special Northern Cyprus courtesy ensign.

There are a number of attractive anchorages along the coast to the east of Girne.

REPUBLIC OF CYPRUS

The notes in the following sections refer only to the Republic of Cyprus.

MAJOR HARBOURS AND MARINAS

There are full marina facilities at Larnaca, close to the centre of the town.

At Limassol mooring facilities for yachts are available at the old harbour which ceased commercial shipping operations in 1974. This yacht harbour is situated in the centre of Limassol. There is also a marina at Limassol St. Raphael, a few kilometres away to the east. This is considered to be the best equipped marina.

Paphos, on the west coast of the island, is a picturesque harbour which is presently under development.

The marinas are crowded and reservation 6-12 months in advance is essential for any stay of over 30 days. Fees have recently been considerably increased.

OTHER INFORMATION

The unit of currency is the Cyprus pound (CYP) divided into 100 cents. Cyprus money is readily accepted in the Turkish area but the Republic of Cyprus will not accept Turkish lira.
Tel. code from the UK: 00 357
Tel. code to the UK: 00 44

During the summer all shops close from 1300 to 1600 and all government offices close for the day at 1330. Bank opening hours are 0830-1200 Monday to Saturday.

ENTRY BY SEA

No yacht may enter the Republic of Cyprus through Northern Cyprus ports or touch at any point on the area controlled by Turkey. According to the Laws of the Republic of Cyprus, entry into the Turkish controlled areas of the island is illegal. Vessels entering those ports are liable to be arrested when within the waters of ports under the control of the Cyprus Government. Entries are closely monitored and a fine of up to 10,000 Cyprus pounds and/ or up to 6 months imprisonment is imposed on any transgressor. All yachts must clear in and out of each port. Landing cards are issued together with form C104 (temporary importation), this form is issued for 12 months and entitles the holder to buy equipment duty free. A total of 3 years temporary importation is allowed before duty must be paid.

When entering Cypriot waters a yacht should fly the Cyprus flag.

Cyprus Radio maintains continuous listening watch on VHF 16 and 26.

It is advised that, unless approaching a port of entry, vessels should maintain a distance of 500m offshore by day and 1,000m by night.

PORTS OF ENTRY
Limassol, Larnaca, Paphos, St. Raphael Marina.

CUSTOMS
Remain on board until clearance has been given by the Marina Attendant, Marine Police, Customs Officer, Immigration Officer and Health Inspector. Passports will be retained by Immigration. A Form C104, valid for 12 months, is issued by Customs.

DUTIABLE STORES
Consumable stores are available 24 hours prior to departure, spirits being limited to one case per person.

Duty free tobacco and liquor on board should be declared on entry and may be removed and retained by the Customs until departure when it will be returned. Duty free tobacco and liquor may be obtained in all ports, where there are bonded stores.

TEMPORARY IMPORTATION
Yachts are welcomed to Cyprus and formalities are simple. They may visit Cyprus for a period of up to one year. For longer stays Customs authority must be obtained and this is normally granted up to a total of three years, any number of visits being cumulative.

DOCUMENTATION

DOCUMENTATION OF VESSEL
Ship's registration papers, which should be presented to the port authorities at the port of entry. Evidence of insurance may be requested.

DOCUMENTATION OF CREW
Valid passports. Crew lists (5 copies) should be made available at the port of entry. Marinas require two passport photos of each adult for the Marina Entry Permit (issued free).

CHARTERING
Contact one of the marinas or JMP Luxury Yacht Cruises, PO Box 4875, Nicosia, Cyprus.

FUEL AND STORES
Good facilities are available at Limassol and Larnaca including diesel. There is a travel-lift at Larnaca.

WEATHER FORECASTS
Only from coastal radio stations or Greek National broadcasts (see Greek section).

Good Navtex forecasts can be received from Limnos, Iraklion and Cyprus.

PUBLICATIONS
BA charts -2074 Cyprus -775 Paphos -776 Kyrenia -796 NE Coast - 850 Limassol 851 Larnaca-Famagusta.
Admiralty Sailing Directions, Mediterranean Pilot Vol V.
The Eastern Mediterranean *Denham.*
Turkish Waters Pilot and Cyprus *Heikell* (Imray) 1997.

USEFUL ADDRESSES
High Commission of the Republic of Cyprus, 93 Park Street, London W1 Tel: 0171 499 8272

Cyprus Tourist Office, 213 Regent Street, London W1R 8DA Tel: 0171 734 2593/9822

Thesea Savva (Admiralty Chart Agents), 118 Franklin Roosevelt Avenue, Limassol, Cyprus.

Larnaca Marina, Tel: 357 653110/653113, Fax: 357 624110.

Cyprus Tourist Office, Nicosia Tel: 357 2 337715

Limassol Marina Tel: 357 532 1100, Fax: 357 532 9208.

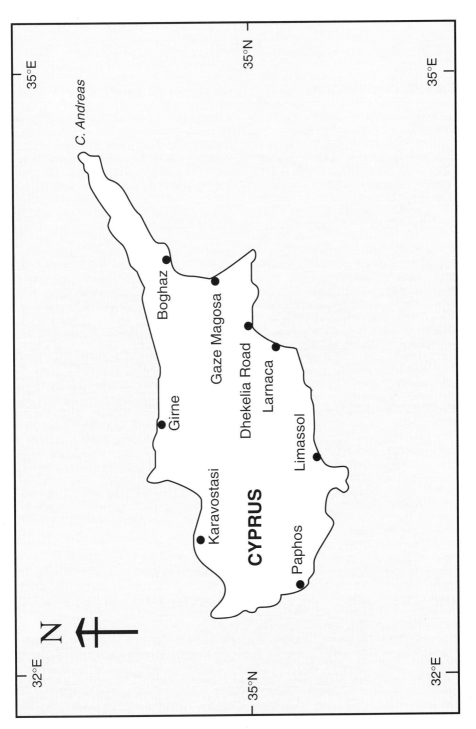

11
TURKEY

GENERAL INFORMATION

Turkey enjoys a variety of climates from the temperate Black Sea region to the continental climate of the interior and the Mediterranean climate of the Aegean and Mediterranean coastal regions. The coastline of Turkey's four seas is more than 4,000M in length.

Apart from the peak holiday period of July and August, it is not difficult to find quiet and secure anchorages on what is one of the best cruising grounds in the Mediterranean.

CRUISING AREAS

The Lycian coast, from Marmaris east to Antalya (about 180 miles).

The Carian coast, from Bodrum south and east to Marmaris, including the Gulf of Gokova and the Datca Peninsula (about 120 miles).

The Ionian coast, from Kusadasi south to Bodrum, including the Gulf of Gulluk (about 80 miles).

The Aeolian coast, from Ayvalik south to Kusadasi (about 180 miles).

From Istanbul south to Ayvalik, including the Sea of Marmara and the Dardanelles (about 220 miles).

MAJOR HARBOURS AND MARINAS

There are excellent marinas where a yacht may be left unattended including Ataköy (Istanbul), Kusadasi, Bodrum, Marmaris, Kemer and Setur (Antalya).

OTHER INFORMATION

The Turkish courtesy flag should be flown at all times, and it should be in good condition.

It is best to avoid zig-zagging between Turkish and Greek waters as this may be misinterpreted.

The coast is under surveillance and visitors should refrain from removing any antiquities from the coast or coastal waters, as the penalty is the confiscation of the yacht.

Although holding tanks are not yet compulsory for private yachts they are a necessity, as even tooth cleaning water is considered an illegal discharge. One yacht was fined £1,000 recently for discharging in harbour, and elsewhere another was confiscated, because the fine was more than the boat was worth. You are in tideless waters and often anchored in places where you want to swim. Although the rules are harshly applied they are sensible. The fines are termed 'voluntary contributions to the civic fund', the alternative is for the boat to be impounded.

There are no facilities anywhere to have holding tanks pumped out from shore and when you need to pump out, you should proceed at least six miles to sea.

Local boats pump out when 300 metres offshore. Charter yachts must have holding tanks, private yachts do not have to have them but there are restrictions on sewage discharge in some harbours, and in all marinas. In particular Bodrum, Bozburon, Gocek (Town Quay), Kalkan, Kas.

The unit of currency is the Turkish lira. There is no limit to the amount of foreign currency that may be brought into Turkey. The exchange slips for the conversion of foreign currency should be kept, they may be required when reconverting Turkish lira back into foreign currency and when taking souvenirs out of the country (to prove that they have been purchased with legally exchanged foreign currency). No more than $5000 worth of Turkish currency may be bought into or taken out of the country. Inflation is very high. Do not cash more than is immediately required.

Banking hours are 0830-1200 and 1300-1700 (not Sat or Sun).

Tel. code from the UK: 00 90
Tel. code to the UK: 00 44

ENTRY BY SEA

The Q flag should be hoisted.

PORTS OF ENTRY

Yachts should enter at a recognised port of entry. These are: Canakkak, Bandirma, Istanbul, Ayvalik, Dikili, Datça, Marmaris, Bodrum, Fethiye, Kas, Kemer, Antalya, Alanya, Tasucu, (Silifke), Mersin, Iskenderun, Finaike,

Samsun, Trabzon, Hopa, Rize, Giresun, Ordu, Smop, Inebolu, Bartir, Zonguldak, Ereguli, Derince, Gemlik, Mundanya, Tokirdag, Akçay, Izmir, Cesme, Kusadasi, Güllok, Anamar, Bozyazi and Botac-Adana.

CUSTOMS

Upon arrival a transit log, valid for 3 months, is purchased from Customs or the marina office. Costing US$30, this must be paid for in hard currency, or proof obtained from the bank that currency has been exchanged.

The transit log contains details of the yacht, crew and ports to be visited. It is not necessary to list every port en route. It is required even if the yacht is to be left at the port of arrival. The transit log will be signed and stamped by the Harbour Master, Health Officer, Customs, Customs Patrol and Passport Police. The yacht's details may be entered in the skipper's passport and must be deleted by Customs before the skipper can leave the country, even if the yacht is left in Turkey. Departure from Turkish waters requires similar clearance from the various authorities before handing in the transit log. The transit log will be cancelled and re-issued in the event of crew changes or re-placement of the person who has completed the log.

Transit logs may be inspected at any harbour or by Customs patrols. The regulations are set out below:

All ports and harbours that may be visited and are beyond final destination should be listed on the transit log. Some Coastguard crews are very particular.

ARTICLE 46

"Foreigners entering Turkey on board their yachts may leave their vessels at a licensed marina for a period of up to two years for winter lay-up, repair and maintenance purposes, and leave the country by other means. Under such circumstances they should apply to the Customs Authorities with a document obtained from the marina manager, and the necessary entries will be made in their passports. The yacht owner may not, under any circumstances, transfer or lend his vessel, while left in Turkey, to a third party or institution.

Yachts left in this manner may stay in Turkey for a period of up to five years without any additional formalities, on condition that the yacht owner utilises his/her vessel once every two years. At the end of this five year period the Ministry of Culture and Tourism holds the authority to extend it further."

ARTICLE 47

"Foreign flagged private yachts coming from foreign harbours, or having wintered in Turkey are allowed to sail in or between Turkish ports, providing that the yacht owner is on board the vessel.

Foreign flagged private yachts with more than one owner, or those owned by clubs or associations may only be used by four different individual owners.

The owners or crew members of private yachts entering Turkish ports are not considered as seamen and may not benefit from the rights given to them, even if they operate such vessels. Guests of Turkish or foreign nationality, recruited crew members and yachtsmen operating rented yachts without crew are also of the same status and may not be considered as seamen and benefit from seamen's rights.

The activities of foreign flagged commercial tourist yachts, which are registered with the Ministry are not regarded as commercial passenger transportation. However, it is forbidden for those yachts to engage in commercial passenger transportation within or between Turkish ports.

Foreign flagged commercial tourist yachts are not allowed to transport passengers on a scheduled or unscheduled basis from a foreign port for the purpose of organising excursions between Turkish ports.

Foreign flagged commercial yachts and foreign-flagged private yachts without their owner on board are required to pay a certain fee at their first port of entry according to the length of the yacht, in order to travel to a second Turkish port.

The fee, valid for one-way travel on a designated schedule, should be paid in one of the convertible foreign currencies, or in an equivalent amount in Turkish lira, upon receipt of the transit log from the first port of entry.

Length of Vessel/Fee
0-10m (inclusive) US$400
10-15m US$600
15-25m US$800
25m and over US$1200

ENTRY BY ROAD

Automobiles, minibuses, caravans, towed sea craft, motorcycles and bicycles can be brought into Turkey for up to three months without a *carnet de passage* or *triptique*. The vehicle is simply registered in the owner's passport and this registration is cancelled when the owner leaves the country. It is not possible to have a car and a boat on one passport unless the boat is towed by the car. For stays longer than three months it is necessary to apply to the Turkish Touring and Automobile Club for a *triptique*, otherwise the vehicle must leave and re-enter the country at the end of three months. If a tourist wishes to visit another country from Turkey without his car he should take the car to the nearest Customs Authority (Gumruk Mudurlugu) so that the registration of the car in his passport may be cancelled and the car kept in a customs area. Drivers need a three-sectioned driving licence or an international driving licence.

Insurance. A motorist should have either:

a) Green Card International Insurance, endorsed for Turkish territory both in Europe and Asia, or

b) Turkish third party insurance, which can be obtained from any of the insurance agencies at the frontier ports.

In case of an accident – whether or not persons are injured, the police should be notified as a report is essential.

DOCUMENTATION

DOCUMENTATION OF VESSEL

Ship's registration papers, Certificate of Insurance, Ship's Radio Licence.

DOCUMENTATION OF CREW

Valid passports. International Certificate of Competence is required for skippers. Visas are required for UK citizens and are valid for one visit only, they can be purchased from the Turkish Embassy or Consulate or on arrival, a fee of £10 is payable in sterling.

CHARTERING

Crewed yachts based on traditional local design (gulets) are available at a number of ports for charter. With modest sail area and powerful diesel, they are very suitable for local conditions. Bareboat and skippered yachts are also widely available for charter. There are also numerous UK based charterers who advertise in yachting magazines.

FUEL, STORES AND REPAIRS

Spares may be difficult to obtain outside Istanbul and Marmaris, and considerable delays may be incurred in importing them. Antifoulings and general chandlery are available at the major marinas. Engine repairs and most general repairs (but not electronics) can be carried out at the major marinas. Atakoy, Kusadasi, Kemer, Setur and Marmaris have travel-lifts. Diesel and water are readily available at most harbours. Camping Gaz is very difficult to find, but Turkish Ipragas has identical fittings and is obtainable everywhere. General provisions, fruit and vegetables are in good supply, as is fresh meat and fish. Few frozen foods are on sale, and a limited range of tinned goods; however the abundance of fresh foods more than compensates for this.

NAVIGATIONAL AIDS

Buoyage and lights are sparse. Hazards are not necessarily marked, and cruising in these waters requires careful study of charts and pilot.

WEATHER FORECASTS

The Greek national radio and coastal radio stations cover Turkish waters.

There is good reception of Navtex forecasts from Iraklion, Limnos and Cyprus. Some coast radio stations (eg Antalya) carry weather bulletins in Turkish and English.

PUBLICATIONS

BA charts for the coast are suitable, but have not been surveyed recently; Turkish charts are also available.

Admiralty Sailing Directions
Black Sea Pilot
Mediterranean Pilot Vol IV
Mediterranean Pilot Vol V
Turkish Waters Pilot *Heikell* (Imray).
The Ionian Islands to the Anatolian Coast *Denham* (Murray)
Turkey's Turquoise Coast *Heikell* (NET)
Turkey – A Travel Survival Kit *Brosnahan* (Lonely Planet)

USEFUL ADDRESSES

Turkish Embassy, 43 Belgrave Square, London SW1 Tel: 0171 393 0202

Turkish Tourist Office, 170/173 Piccadilly, London W1V 9DD Tel: 0171 629 7771 Fax: 0171 491 0773

Turkish Maritime Lines, London Sunquest Holidays Ltd, 23 Princes Street, London W1R 7RG Tel: 0171 499 9992 Fax: 0171 499 9995

Minister of Tourism, Inonu Bul. No5 Bahcelievler, Ankara Tel: 0090 10312 Fax: 0090 10312 213 6887

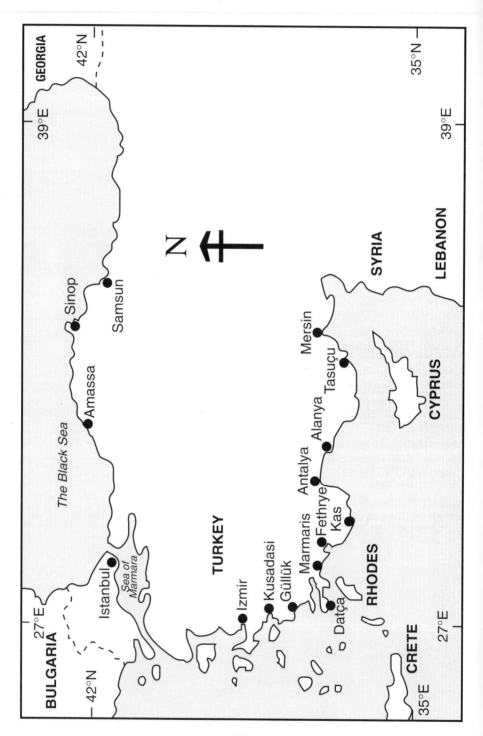

12
THE BLACK SEA

This area is not difficult to reach from the Aegean, and is the natural sequel to a visit to Istanbul, where plentiful stores can and should be taken on board. The passage northwards up the Bosphorus is most rewarding and easily completed in a day; there is a good overnight anchorage at Poyraz on the east bank at the northern end of the Bosphorus.

Since the opening of the Main-Donau Canal, it is also possible to reach the Black Sea via the inland waterways of Europe. (See chapter 21). There is access from the Black Sea to the Russian Inland Waterways which are now open to pleasure craft.

GPS and RDF are the only navigational aids in the Black Sea.

Countries bordering the Black Sea, starting from the west bank of the Bosphorus, are Turkey, Bulgaria, Romania, Ukraine, Russia, Georgia and back to Turkey.

BULGARIA

The main ports are Burgas and Varna. Visiting yachtsmen will need visas, obtainable from the Bulgarian Embassy in London or Istanbul or on entry. British yachtsmen have visited Bulgaria in recent years and experienced no difficulty. Usual ships's papers will be required. Certificates of Competence have been demanded.

Yachts visiting Bulgaria in recent years have found it advisable to clear in and out of Varna, so as to be able to visit other harbours, not possible apparently if first visiting Burgas, which in any case is not recommended for yachts.

ROMANIA

Romania has only a short coastline south of the Danube Delta, and the principal port is Constanta. There is a major commercial area of docks which should not be entered by a visiting yacht. There is a separate pleasure port below the old town where a yacht can lie alongside the quay. Customs officers will come to the yacht; the usual ship's papers are required and visas, which are available from the Romanian Embassy in London or on entry.

Travel within Romania is unrestricted and English and French are widely spoken.

There is only one harbour, at Mangaalya. Yachts may cruise the Danube Delta but berthing facilities are minimal.

UKRAINE, RUSSIA AND GEORGIA

Ukraine includes the port of Odessa and the Crimean Peninsula, including ports such as Yalta and Kereh. The coastline of the Sea of Azor is Russian, and the eastern shores of the Black Sea are mainly Georgian.

NORTHERN COAST OF TURKEY

This area is not much visited by yachts and there are no marinas. However there are many harbours where a yacht can find shelter. The Black Sea coast of Turkey has not been affected by tourism. The natural hospitality of the Turks and the unspoiled nature of the coast suggest this is a promising cruising ground. The formalities are as for the rest of Turkey (see chapter 11). Many yachts have visited this area of late and have reported favourably upon it.

PUBLICATIONS

Admiralty Sailing Directions Black Sea
Admiralty Radio Signals

USEFUL ADDRESSES

Romanian Embassy, 4 Palace Green, London W8 4QD Tel: 0171 937 9666
Romanian Tourist Office, 17 Nottingham Street, London W1 Tel: 0171 224 3692
Bulgarian Embassy, 188 Queen's Gate, London SW7 Tel: 0171 584 9400
Bulgarian Tourist Office, 18 Princes Street, London W1 Tel: 0171 499 6988
Russian Embassy, 5 Kensington Palace Gardens, London W1 Tel: 0171 229 8027
Russian Consulate 24 hour visa information line Tel: 0891 171271
Ukrainian Embassy 60 Holland Park, London W11 Tel: 0171 727 6312
Georgia Embassy 3 Harton Place, Kensington, London W8 4LZ
Tel: 0171 937 8233

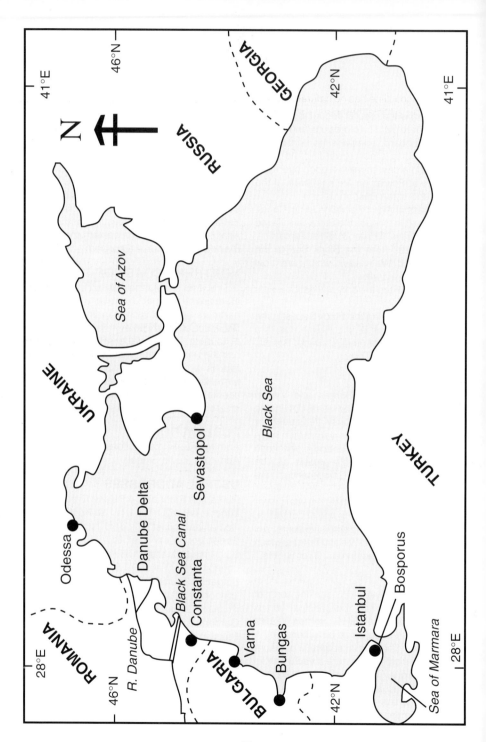

13
SYRIA

The short coastline has no natural harbours and only four artificial harbours – at Latakia, Baniyas, Tartous and Ruad. These are purely commercial ports without facilities for yachts. Nor is there any provision for yachts in the scale of fees for berthing, port services, etc. As a result, a visiting yacht is likely to be charged several hundred dollars for a stay of a few days, without water, electricity or any other facility.

Yachts that have been able to connect to the mains electricity have reported problems due to voltage not being as publicised. Care is required.

The language is Arabic, but French and to some extent English are widely understood.

The unit of currency is the Syrian pound (S£) divided into 100 piastres.

US $ are commonly used and are extremely useful.

Tel. code from the UK: 00 963
Tel. code to the UK: 00 44

ENTRY BY SEA

Yachts may not visit Syria if Israeli stamps are on crew passports.

Arrival should be made preferably at Latokia, in daylight, and at 90º to the coast. ETA must be reported when 12 miles west of the port. Visiting yachts are not permitted to cruise along the coast and navigation at night is not recommended in view of the risk of being taken for a hostile vessel.

Formalities have been reported as complicated. Yachts planning to visit Syria are recommended to try and arrange for the services of a local agent beforehand.

DOCUMENTATION OF CREW

Valid passports and visas.

Visa can be obtained in London or on arrival in which case extra passport photographs will be required. Passports should be carried at all times when ashore since security checks are frequent.

An international driving licence is required if driving in Syria.

PUBLICATIONS

BA charts numbers 2632 and 2633 cover the Syrian coast; 1036 and 2796 give harbour plans.

Admiralty Sailing Directions
Mediterranean Pilot Vol V

USEFUL ADDRESSES

The Syrian Embassy, 8 Belgrave Square, London SW1 Tel: 0171 245 9012

There is no Syrian Tourist Office in London, but the Syrian Interest Section at the above address may help.

14
LEBANON

GENERAL INFORMATION

Although there is still tension in the border area between Lebanon and Israel, Lebanon is essentially a peaceful country with good facilities for visiting yachtsmen, at least at Jounieh, a relatively affluent suburb of Beirut.

Jounieh Marina is modern, well equipped and hospitable. The nearby town has good shopping and banking facilities, and the interior of the country has great scenic variety and historic interest.

French and (to a lesser extent) English are widely spoken.

The unit of currency is the Lebanese pound.

Tel. code from the UK: 00 961

Tel. code to the UK: 00 44

Telephone calls to the UK can be made through the operator from the PTT in the town.

US$ notes are acceptable in most shops and restaurants. Other currency is freely exchanged at banks and change shops. Eurocheques are not accepted anywhere. Travellers cheques are grudgingly accepted at some change shops but not at banks.

ENTRY BY SEA

Although Beirut and Tripoli are official ports of entry it is advisable to head first for Jounieh, where foreign yachtsmen are welcomed and where neither formalities nor security represent a problem. The procedure for entry is to contact 'Oscar Charlie' on VHF Ch.11 when 20M offshore on a bearing of 270° from port of entry. Request entry and you will be allocated a clearance number or you can get it in advance by calling the Marina Manager. You should report again at 12M and 6M when this number will be asked for. Yachts arriving from Israel will be denied entry. An Israeli stamp on a crew passport will preclude entry.

On arrival at Jounieh Marina, Customs should be contacted from the fuel berth just inside the entrance, but yachts are usually allocated a berth in the marina and immigration formalities completed in the marina office. There is a fee, about US $75, for Customs and Immigration clearance, but there are no mooring fees for the first three days.

DOCUMENTATION

DOCUMENTATION OF VESSEL

Ship's registration papers.

Letter of authority if the owner is not aboard.

DOCUMENTATION OF CREW

Valid passports, and visas which can be obtained on arrival.

Crew list.

FUEL, STORES AND REPAIRS

Diesel and petrol are available without formality at the fuelling berth just inside the marina entrance.

There is a yacht chandler near the marina gate and several good supermarkets in the town. Cash can be obtained with the more common credit cards through a variety of banks.

WEATHER FORECASTS

Weather forecasts can be obtained daily from the marina office.

PUBLICATIONS

British Admiralty Charts and Sailing Directions are adequate.

USEFUL ADDRESSES

Lebanese Embassy, Consular Section,
21 Kensington Palace Gardens,
London W8 4RA
Tel: 0171 229 7265.

Jounieh Marina
Automobile and Touring Club du Liban,
Jounieh BP115, Lebanon
Tel: 961 9 932 020/640 220
Fax: 961 9 640 579/934 662

15
ISRAEL

GENERAL INFORMATION

Israel's coastal waters have little to offer cruising yachts, but many of those who find themselves at this end of the Mediterranean may want to visit the tourist sites.

MAJOR HARBOURS AND MARINAS

Tel Aviv Marina has excellent security and modern facilities but is somewhat expensive and usually crowded. It also has a very difficult entrance from the sea, and entry should not be attempted with onshore winds in anything other than calm conditions. The marina will provide a pilot without charge if requested by VHF.

The marina at Haifa, within the commercial port area, has fewer facilities but is considerably cheaper. There are new marinas at Hertzlia, Ashdod and Ashkezon. Ashkezon is the port of entry, ideal for boats en route to or from the Red Sea.

There are also harbours at Akko and Jaffa.

OTHER INFORMATION

Tel. code from the UK: 00 972
Tel. code to the UK: 00 44
The unit of currency is the shekel.

Banking hours are 0830-1230 daily except Saturdays and 1600-1700 Sunday, Monday and Tuesday.

ENTRY BY SEA

The Q flag should be flown on approaching Israeli waters.

The coast is patrolled by gunboats and aircraft which intercept all craft approaching their waters. Vessels should report by VHF on Channel 16 to the Israeli Navy when within 50 miles of the coastline. One is advised to listen constantly on Channel 16 while in Israeli waters and be prepared to identify the yacht and report position, course and speed if required. Use callsign 'Israeli Navy', no other callsign is ever answered.

PORTS OF ENTRY

Ports of entry are Haifa, Tel Aviv and Ashdod. In Tel Aviv authorities are situated within the marina but in Haifa they are some distance away.

CUSTOMS

On arrival it is necessary to report to the police. Crew may not leave the yacht until this has been done. Landing cards will often be issued in place of passports which will be returned upon request if needed for bank transactions or booking travel arrangements.

DOCUMENTATION

DOCUMENTATION OF VESSEL

Ship's registration papers.

DOCUMENTATION OF CREW

Valid passports. Visas are not required by British passport holders.

Passports are normally stamped on entry but on request the police will stamp a separate sheet of paper to prevent difficulties when visiting other countries.

FUEL, STORES AND PROVISIONS

The range of goods available in the shops is similar to that found in most western countries, although prices tend to be slightly higher. Fresh produce may be bought more cheaply in the markets. Petrol and diesel can be obtained without difficulty at the fuel berth in Tel Aviv Marina and supplies may be arranged, albeit with somewhat greater difficulty, at the other harbours.

NAVIGATIONAL AIDS

Haifa and Tel Aviv are well lit.

PUBLICATIONS

BA chart number 2634 covers the coast and 1585 and 1591 give harbour plans.
Admiralty Sailing Directions, Mediterranean Pilot Vol V.

USEFUL ADDRESSES

Israeli Embassy, 2 Palace Green, Kensington, London W8 4QB Tel: 0171 957 9500

Israeli National Tourist Office, 18 Great Marlborough Street, London W1V 1AS Tel: 0171 434 3651

The Ministry of Transport – Division of Shipping and Ports, PO Box 33993 Haifa. Tel: 04 520241

Hertzlia Marina Tel: 972 9 565591 Fax: 972 9 565593

Ashkezon Marina Tel: 972 7 733780 Fax: 972 7 733823

16
EGYPT

GENERAL INFORMATION
English and French are widely spoken.

CRUISING AREAS
The Mediterranean coastline consists of a long stretch of sandy beaches. There is very little shelter and the coast is mostly exposed to breakers and northerly winds.

MAJOR HARBOURS AND MARINAS
Alexandria has a western and an eastern harbour, each protected by a breakwater. The eastern harbour is recommended for visiting yachts; it has a designated anchorage area for yachts and small craft, with fairly good holding.

Port Said lies at the northern end of the Suez Canal, and a berth may be found at the Port Fouad Yacht Club or the anchorage nearby. There is very heavy commercial traffic at Port Said.

INLAND WATERWAYS
Suez Canal – the procedure for transiting the Suez Canal is quite complex and very time-consuming unless an agent is employed. The Felix Maritime Agency (Nagib Latif) specialises in assisting foreign yachts to pass through the Canal and operates in accordance with a published price list.

Use of an agent is strongly recommended and this could avoid unpleasant difficulties.

The River Nile – a yacht should only attempt navigation of the Nile subject to the following requirements:
- a strong hull to withstand stone banks and passing barges
- a powerful engine to overcome strong currents
- removable masts
- maximum draft of 1.75m
- reliable echo sounder

OTHER INFORMATION
Tel. code from the UK: 00 20
Tel. code to the UK: 00 44
The unit of currency is the Egyptian pound divided into 100 piastres.

ENTRY BY SEA

PORTS OF ENTRY
Alexandria and Port Said, or Safaya, Hazghada and Suez if arriving via the Red Sea.

CUSTOMS
If an agent is employed, he will normally handle all dealings with the Customs and Immigration authorities. Otherwise, the yacht will be visited by Coastguards and Customs Officials.

Special Customs measures are taken for yachts intending to enter the Nile or the Suez Canal.

DOCUMENTATION

DOCUMENTATION OF VESSEL
Ship's registration papers, Ship's Radio Licence.

The following documents should be obtained at the port of entry:
1. Currency transfer receipt
2. Health Certificate
3. Security permit (for the River Nile)
4. Customs list showing the yacht's equipment.
5. Insurance Policy (for the Suez Canal)

Any or all of these documents should be shown as demanded by the local authorities, when applying for visa renewal or a departure permit.

Six copies of the crew list showing surname, forenames, passport number, status aboard (i.e. crew member) and date of birth.

DOCUMENTATION OF CREW
Valid passport.

Entry into Egypt is open to yachts and yachtsmen of all nationalities. Israelis are permitted provided they carry an entry visa previously obtained from the Egyptian Embassy or Consulate in Israel.

All crew members will require an entry visa, obtainable from Egyptian Embassies and

Consulates abroad, or from local authorities on arrival at any port of entry.

Usually visas are valid for thirty days from the date of issue, an additional fifteen days is permissible provided there are good reasons for the long stay. On expiry, a new visa should be applied for, in which case you may be required to transfer the sum of US$180 per person, or the equivalent, into Egyptian currency. Children under the age of twelve are exempted from the requirements to transfer currency.

Your entry visa must be registered at the main office of Immigration, Passports and Nationality Administration at the port of entry, within seven days of acquisition. Failure to do so will result in a fine.

No restrictions are placed on the amount in cash or travellers' cheques carried or transferred, provided it is declared. The transfer or exchange of currency should be made through banks or their branches in certain first class hotels. You are warned not to deal with the black market, however profitable it may appear.

DEPARTURE REGULATIONS

Yachts departing from Egypt should do so from a port of entry. A departure permit should be applied for from the Coast Guard Authorities. All permits, documents and currency transfer receipts previously obtained on arrival or transfer should be submitted, together with passports and the crew list, to the Authorities. Any changes in the crew members must be entered on the crew list. Yachts should depart as soon as the departure permit is obtained. However, in case of difficulty such as engine trouble, serious damage, foul weather or absence of favourable winds, departure can be postponed for 24 hours. If the departure is delayed for longer than 24 hours then you will have to apply for a fresh departure permit.

PUBLICATIONS

BA charts numbers 3356, 2574 and 2573 cover the coast.

Numbers 3325, 3326, 3119, 243, 2681 and 2578 provide harbour approaches and plans; 234 and 233 are required for the Suez Canal and approach.

Admiralty Sailing Directions:
Mediterranean Pilot Vol V
Red Sea and Indian Ocean Cruising Guide *Lucas* (Imray)
Egypt for Yachtsmen from the Egyptian Tourist Information Office.

USEFUL ADDRESSES

Arabic Republic of Egypt Embassy (Consular Affairs), 2 Lowndes Street, London SW1X 9ET Tel: 0171 235 9777

Egypt Tourist Information Office, 168 Piccadilly, London W1 Tel: 0171 493 5282

Egyptair, 29 Picadilly, London W1 Tel: 0171 437 6309

Centralex Marine Horizon, 10 Mohamed Ahmed El Afify Street, San Stefano, Alexandria, Egypt Tel: 03 586 4939

Felix Maritime Agency, PO Box 618, Port Said, Egypt Tel: 0020 66 244401 Fax: 0020 66 242443

17
LIBYA

The Foreign and Commonwealth Office advises that in spite of the operation of sanctions it is still possible to visit Libya and that there should be no major security problem. As in other strict Muslim countries however, it is important for visitors to avoid giving offence to the local population. It is necessary to exercise great sensitivity for local standards and codes of behaviour. Dress should be modest. There should be no public display of affection between individuals. Pork and alcohol are forbidden. Photography in the vicinity of ports, stations and other public utility installations should be avoided.

The Libyan section of the Saudi Arabian Embassy in London advises that visas should be obtained before arrival. It is unclear, however, whether as in many countries with similar rules, it may be possible for the crews of vessels arriving by sea to be issued with temporary shore passes at the time of arrival.

All vessels navigating in Libyan waters should have serviceable VHF radio equipment and should keep a listening watch on Channel 16 at all times. Port authorities should be contacted on Channel 11, 12 or 16 before arrival, permission is required to move from one Libyan port to another. Movement in Libyan waters is permitted only by day. Refuse and waste water may not be discharged; holding tanks are essential.

Insurance companies may be reluctant to offer cover in this area.

18
ALGERIA

Although the 750M rugged coastline of Algeria has a number of possible ports and fishing harbours, including a marina at Sidi Fredj, near Algiers, the Foreign and Commonwealth Office strongly advises against visiting the country because the political situation is unstable. There have been numerous murders and armed attacks on foreigners in recent times and yachtsmen are advised to avoid calling at Algerian ports or approaching the coast.

19
TUNISIA

GENERAL INFORMATION

Tunisia has some 820M of coastline – 650 of them sandy beaches. As a rule safe berth can be found after a coastal passage of no more than 40 miles. The official language is Arabic, but most Tunisians also speak French.

Tunisia is hotter than countries in the north of the Mediterranean and is pleasantest in the autumn or spring. Winds are reasonably consistent in direction and strength, but in the spring they often blow from the south, carrying sand which will deposit itself all over the decks.

It is reported that care is required with laid up moorings in Monostir Marina due to very strong NW winds which are common in winter.

The crime rate in Tunisia is low. The cost of living is relatively low, half that of London.

Tel. code from the UK: 00 216

Tel. code to the UK: 00 44

The unit of currency is the Tunisian dinar (TND), divided into 1,000 millimes. Dinars may not be imported into Tunisia. Banking hours are Monday to Friday 0800-1100 in the summer and an additional two hours in the afternoon during the winter.

MAJOR HARBOURS AND MARINAS

There are six major marinas:-

Tabarka, which is a fishing harbour with a new marina.

Bizerta, a large commercial harbour near the end of a canal, has a small marina in the outer harbour with guest pontoon.

Sidi Bou Said marina has a travel-lift and limited chandlery.

Tunis, another large commercial port up a canal, has a marina near the entrance at La Goulette, which tends to be full most of the time.

El Kantaoui marina has a travel-lift and visitors berths. It is some distance from shopping facilities although there is a small local supermarket.

Monastir is a large marina with a well run travel-lift. Chandlery suitable for fishing boats is available from hardware shops in the town.

The marina is near the town centre and convenient for the airport.

A marina is under construction at Hammanet South, due for completion in 2001.

In addition to these marinas there are major harbours, including Kelibia, Sousse, Mahdia and Sfax.

ENTRY BY SEA

Yachts must report at an official port of entry to Port Police, Harbour Officers, Customs and Frontier Police who will all study yacht and personal documents and stamp them. All personnel must remain on board until formalities have been completed. Passports will be stamped with a three month entry permit which may be renewed for a further three months. Customs will issue a *manifeste* and the Frontier Police a *Declaration d'Entree*, granting permission to cruise in Tunisian waters for three months. Crew lists may be required both at the initial entry and at subsequent ports of call.

On departure, it is necessary to report to Customs and Frontier Police. If there is no local office, time must be allowed for officials to arrive from the nearest town or airport. The entry documents must be surrendered and passports stamped.

Anchoring along the coast, especially at night, is forbidden without prior authorisation, however short daylight stops appear to be tolerated. Checks are made by patrol craft.

Tunisians are not allowed to board foreign yachts.

PORTS OF ENTRY

Tabarka, Bizerta, Sidi Bou Said, La Goulette, Kelibia, El Kantaoui, Sousse, Monastir, Mahdia, Gabes, Houmt-Souk and Zarzis.

CUSTOMS

Customs will require a list of all valuable equipment carried on the yacht. The export of dinars is strictly forbidden, and exchange receipts should be retained in order to facilitate the sale of surplus dinars on departure.

Antiques may only be exported by permission of the Ministry of Cultural Affairs.

TEMPORARY IMPORTATION

The Tunisian authorities encourage yacht owners to keep their yachts permanently in the country, and the facilities reflect this. Owners leaving their boats in Tunisia to return home by air can obtain a document from Customs which enables them to bring back yacht equipment duty free.

Yachts may be 'immobilised' for the winter by Customs and this period will not count against the 6 months total navigation period. It is reported that to be granted this concession the owner must first have a contract with the relevant marina. Whilst 'immobilised' the yacht may not be moved without the permission of the Harbour Police.

DOCUMENTATION

DOCUMENTATION OF VESSEL

Ship's registration papers. Evidence of ownership of the vessel may be required. In this connection it is important to note that the SSR document on its own does not satisfy this requirement. A bill of sale should also be carried (or a charter party agreement if the yacht is not owned by the persons on board). An insurance certificate, a list of objects of value, and a list of firearms should be carried. A crew list may be required at each port of call.

DOCUMENTATION OF CREW

Valid passports.

An International Certificate of Competence is advisable. There are no restrictions on crew changes provided these are notified.

Visa needed after three month stay.

Non-EU Citizens may require a visa and they should enquire at the Tunisian Embassy in London beforehand.

CHARTERING

The Tunisian National Tourist Office can supply details of chartering facilities. Cruising yachts and catamarans can be chartered from Tunisia Yachting Loisirs at Monastir. Le Club Nautique de Sidi Bou Said (Tel: 270 689) will advise on local sailing and water skiing.

FUEL AND STORES

Fuel is cheaper than in many Mediterranean countries and there are fuel berths at all the main marinas. Water is usually available, and it is possible to have Camping Gaz bottles refilled at Sidi Bou Said, El Kantaoui and Monastir. It is also possible to use Tunisian gas bottles with a Camping Gaz installation. General stores are available in markets and supermarkets. Wine and beer can be obtained, spirits are expensive.

NAVIGATIONAL AIDS

There is good buoyage around major ports. For RDF stations see Mediterranean Almanac (Imray).

WEATHER FORECASTS

Weather forecasts may be obtained from the Harbour Master or by contacting the marine weather centre at the coastal ports of La Goulette, Sfax, Mahdia or Bizerta.

A shipping forecast (in French) is broadcast by Tunis Radio on 1768.4kHz. Forecasts can also be received from Lampadusa (in English and Italian) on 1876kHz and from Malta (in English) on 2624.8kHz.

PUBLICATIONS

BA charts are adequate for cruising in Tunisia. French charts are more detailed and more up to date.
Admiralty Sailing Directions:
Mediterranean Pilot Vol 1
Guide to Tunisia *Maurice* (McMillan Graham)
North Africa *RCC* (Imray)
Rough Guide to Tunisia (Penguin)

USEFUL ADDRESSES

Tunisian Embassy, 29 Prince's Gate, London SW7 1QG Tel: 0171 584 8117

Tunisian National Tourist Office, 77a Wigmore Street, London W1H 9LJ Tel: 0171 224 5561

Tunisian National Tourist Office,
1 Av. Mohamed V, Tunis Tel: 341 077

Tunisia Yachting Loisirs, Monastir

20
MOROCCO

GENERAL INFORMATION
From the Algerian frontier to the Straits of Gibraltar the sandy coast extends for some 250M with rocky promontories of which Cabo Tres Forcas is the most notable. The vast range of the Rif Mountains rise above the frequent low-lying mists which can develop rapidly into dense fogs.

DRUGS
It should be noted that the Moroccan authorities are waging a major campaign against drug smuggling. Yachts are automatically suspect and may be searched at any time. It is best to avoid anchoring or night passages along the coast.

Anchoring is not normally allowed near harbours.

OTHER INFORMATION
Tel. code from the UK: 00 212
Tel. code to the UK: 00 44
The unit of currency is the dirham (Dh), divided into 100 centimes. Dirhams may not be exported.

Ferries ply from Algeciras to Ceuta and Tangier.

MAJOR HARBOURS AND MARINAS
There are large harbours at Tangier Al Hoceima and the Spanish enclaves of Ceuta and Melilla and smaller ones at El Jebha, Ras el Ma and M'Diq (which may not be open for yachts). There are marinas at Restinga Smir and Kabila.

ENTRY BY SEA
There are no defined ports of entry but yachts are required to report to both Customs and Immigration authorities on arrival and prior to departure. Entry and clearance formalities are in fact required at all ports visited. Customs offices exist everywhere except in the smallest harbours and Port police will be found throughout.

The Q flag should be hoisted when entering Moroccan waters.

FUEL AND STORES
There are no facilities for embarking duty-free stores. Fuel and water are usually available. Camping Gaz can be obtained in Ceuta and Melilla.

TEMPORARY IMPORTATION
An initial period of three months is permitted.

DOCUMENTATION

DOCUMENTATION OF VESSEL
Ship's registration papers.

DOCUMENTATION OF CREW
Valid passports, but no visas. Crew changes are not restricted. There are reports of entry being refused if Israeli stamps are on crew passports.

PUBLICATIONS
BA charts Numbers 773 and 2437 cover the coast, and 580 gives harbour plans.
Admiralty Sailing Directions:
Mediterranean Pilot Vol I
North African Pilot *von Riju* (RCC/Imray)

USEFUL ADDRESSES
Moroccan Embassy, 49 Queens Gate Gardens, London SW7 5NE
Tel: 0171 581 5001

Moroccan National Tourist Office, 205 Regent Street, London W1R 7DE
Tel: 0171 437 0073 Fax: 0171 734 8172

21
RHINE-DANUBE LINK

GENERAL INFORMATION

Since the opening of the Main-Donau Canal in September 1992, a major new route from western Europe to the Black Sea and the eastern Mediterranean has been available for yachts drawing under 1.8m and with masts unstepped.

For yachts not capable of cruising at more than 6-7 knots the route leads from England via the French canals to Strasbourg, down the Rhine to Frankfurt, up the Main and through the Main-Donau Canal to join the Danube at Kelheim. From Kelheim the rest of the journey is downstream on the Danube until the Black Sea is reached via the canal link near Constanta in Romania.

Vessels with enough power to cruise at 10 knots can also consider reaching the Main by travelling upstream in the Rhine, either from the Mosel or all the way from Holland. The Main is completely canalised and currents are negligible. The Danube, although canalised, is quite fast-flowing especially when it is in flood. Vessels without a great deal of engine power should avoid such times, even for a downstream passage, as harbour entry manoeuvres can be dangerous when the current is strong. Similarly, upstream passages are likely to be impracticable at any time for slow-moving vessels.

The Danube is an international waterway, and the formalities required are few. It is necessary, however, for each crew member to obtain a transit visa for the passage through the Serbian section of the river. This can be done, without having to produce an invitation, either in London or Budapest. Romanian visas are needed and these should preferably be obtained before starting the journey.

DOCUMENTATION

DOCUMENTATION OF VESSEL

Ship's registration papers, Ship's Radio Licence and insurance should be carried. Rhine regulations must be carried when on the Rhine.

Vessels longer than 20 metres will probably have to comply completely with local vessel requirements. These are likely to be to full commercial specifications and are contained in the Règlement de visite. All vessels must comply with the Règlement de Police.

DOCUMENTATION OF CREW

Valid passports, visas where appropriate (see above), and Certificates of Competence (ICC) are necessary. Vessels of more than 15 metres length must carry a Rhine pilot when navigating the Rhine and a Danube pilot in Austria.

A Rhine sportsboat patent (licence) is available for vessels 15-25 metres but this demands 16 recent voyages on that part of the river for which the licence is issued. This is therefore only available to locals. No such licence exists in Austria.

PUBLICATIONS

The Danube – A River Guide *Heikell* (Imray)
The RYA Book of EuroRegs - available from the RYA

USEFUL ADDRESSES

Hungarian Embassy (Consulate & Visa Section), 35 Eaton Place,
London SW1X 8BY Tel: 0171 235 2664

Romanian Consulate, 4 Palace Green,
London W8 Tel: 0171 937 9666

Commission Centrale pour la Navigation du Rhin, 2 place de la Republique 67082 Strasbourg Cedex
Tel:+03 88 52 20 10 Fax: +03 88 32 10 72